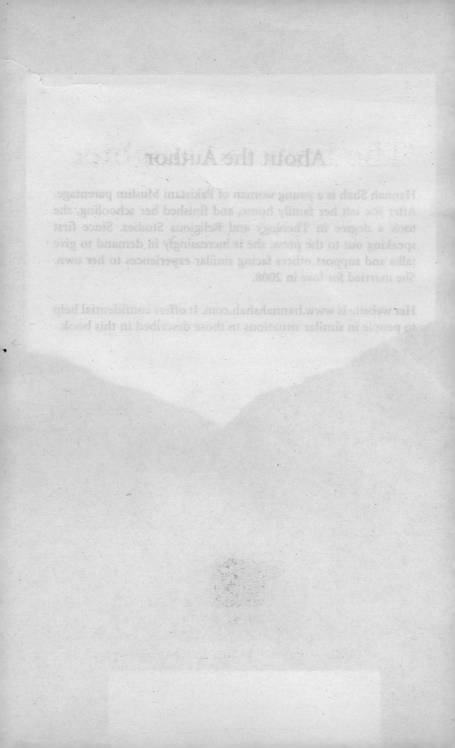

The Imam's Daughter

Hannah Shah

RIDER

London • Sydney • Auckland • Johannesburg

1 3 5 7 9 10 8 6 4 2

Published in 2009 by Rider, an imprint of Ebury Publishing
This edition published by Rider in 2010

Ebury publishing is a Random House Group company

Copyright © Hannah Shah 2009

Hannah Shah has asserted her right to be identified as the author of this work
in accordance with the Copyright, Designs and Patents Act 1988

The Random House Group Limited Reg. No. 954009

Addresses for ~~companies within the Random House Group can~~ be found at

A CIP catal~~ogue record for this book is available from the Britis~~h Library

The Rand~~om House Group supports the Forest Stew~~ardship
Council (FSC~~), the leading international forest certification organ~~isation. All
our titles tha~~t are printed on Greenpeace-approved FSC-certified~~ paper carry
the F~~SC logo. Our paper procurement policy can be viewe~~d at

FSC www.fsc.org Cert no. TT-COC-2139
© 1996 Forest Stewardship Council

Typeset by SX Composing DTP, Rayleigh, Essex
Printed and bound in Great Britain by CPI Cox & Wyman, Reading, RG1 8EX

ISBN 9781846041488

To buy books by your favourite authors and register for offers visit
www.rbooks.co.uk

The author would like to thank the following for permission to use copyright
material: HarperCollins Publishers for the excerpt from *The Invitation* by
Oriah Mountain Dreamer (1999) and Puffin, an imprint of Penguin Books,
for verses quoted from *Please Mrs Butler* by Allan Ahlberg (1984). Every effort
has been made to trace and credit all copyright holders but if any have been
inadvertently overlooked the author and publisher will be pleased to make the
necessary arrangements at the first opportunity.

Contents

Acknowledgements

Special thanks to my literary agents in the UK and the USA, for your faith and belief that mine was a story that should be told. Very special thanks to Josephine Tait, a religious freedom campaigner whose advice, friendship and help has proven invaluable. Thanks to Tom, for being an amazing husband and partner for life. Thanks to Lizzy and Mike, and family, who've given me a safe place to grow and to heal. Thanks to Felicity and James, for providing me with a way out and a gateway into the future.

Author's Note

This is a true story, and it happened to me between the year of my birth and the present day. Some names, details about people and places and place locations (notably in relation to my family) and details of all educational establishments have been changed, to protect my identity and guard against potential reprisals, and to protect the identity of others in my story who may be vulnerable. I am aware of the nature of such risks, but I am equally determined that mine is a story that should be told. For clarification, there is no such town as Bermford – the location of the first sixteen years of my life – in England, and I have chosen to create a location that does not exist to protect myself and others from being identified, and from reprisals. Likewise, Hannah Shah is a pseudonym.

This book is my own, personal story. It deals with the way that Islam was practised within my own community as I witnessed it when I was growing up. It is worth pointing out that there are many Muslims in Britain and around the world who have had only good experiences of growing up within their faith, including women who are free to live full, independent and liberated lives and Imams who practise lawfully and have an extremely positive influence on their communities. This book is in no way a denigration of Islam generally. It is a personal account of my own life experiences.

Dedicated to 'My Little Chicken' – you
are precious and I love you.
'I pray that you will be rooted and
established in love.'
Ephesians 4:17

H.S.

For Mum.

The ultimate weakness of violence is that it is a descending spiral, begetting the very thing it seeks to destroy. Instead of diminishing evil, it multiplies it. Through violence you may murder the liar, but you cannot murder the lie. Through violence you may murder the hater, but you do not murder hate. So it goes. Returning violence for violence multiplies violence, adding deeper darkness to a night already devoid of stars. Darkness cannot drive out darkness: only light can do that. Hate cannot drive out hate: only love can.

Dr Martin Luther King, Jr

Believe nothing, O monks, merely because you have been told it.

Or because it is traditional, or because you yourselves have imagined it.

Do not believe what your teacher tells you merely out of respect for the teacher.

But whatsoever you find to be conducive to the good, the benefit and welfare of all beings – that doctrine believe and cling to and take it as your guide.

Gautama Buddha

The whole problem with the world is that fools and fanatics are always so certain of themselves, and wiser people so full of doubt.

Bertrand Russell

One word frees us of all the weight and pain of life:
that word is *love*.

Sophocles

And now, these three continue forever:
Faith, hope and love,
And the greatest of these is love.

1 Corinthians 13:13

Chapter One

My Street

Did you ever play 'monsters under the stairs'? I guess a lot of kids did when they were little. It's Dad, of course – you know it's your dad. But you pretend it's not. You pretend not to know that he's the monster, just to make it a little more scary, just to justify your running, screaming, crying, head-over-heels laughter.

You're off to bed, and Mum doesn't quite approve. She's right behind you, gentle hands ushering you up the stairs. She thinks Dad's monster act will give you nightmares. You think that's rubbish. You love it. You secretly hope tonight's the night. Tonight Dad's going to spring out and give you a great big monster surprise.

You pause on the third step of the staircase.

'Dad, you're not going to be a monster tonight, are you?' Secretly, you're praying that he will. 'Not a monster under the stairs.'

Then, suddenly: 'Roooaarrrr! Roooaaarrr! ROOOAARRR!'

He's there! It's him! It's so much fun and so deliciously, wonderfully *scary*. What do you do? Rush up the staircase and jump into bed, but risk getting got by the monster in the process? Or dash back down again into your mother's ever so patient, protective arms?

It's Dad with a lamp held in front of his face, all silly expressions and shadows in the darkness beneath you. It's Dad, growling like a scary monster, yet all the while trying to choke down his gurgling laughter. It's Dad, fingers curled like a dragon's talons, grabbing for your skinny, pyjama-clad legs, as you, a little

1

five-year-old child, scream and laugh and play act scared and try to get up to bed before he can get you.

It's Dad with a pillow on his head, Dad standing on a chair to make himself look huge, Dad with his fingers in his mouth doing a wide-mouthed-frog-monster-scream at you, and all the while trying to hide the fun and the love in his eyes. It's Dad. It's only Dad. It's just your silly, adoring, ever so indulgent father.

It's not that scary really 'cause it's only Dad.

It's not that scary really, because you never had a dad like mine for your father. It's never been Dad savagely tugging at the rope to bind you tighter on the cold bare floor. It's never been Dad with his robe pulled up, his knuckles dragging you towards him by your hair. It's never been Dad forcing your hand or your face nearer and nearer. It's never been Dad tearing at your clothing, eyes filled with loathing and lust.

It's never been that. *Never that.* Or at least I pray it hasn't been. For I'd never wish my childhood on my worst enemies.

Imagine for one moment that the monsters-under-the-stairs game is for real. Imagine your father is the beast, more terrifying and dark than your childish mind could ever have made him. Imagine living the monsters-under-the-stairs game for real.

Your father is the monster under the stairs, and you are his helpless child victim.

How can I write this so that it doesn't read like scenes from a horror movie? Perhaps I can't. All I can do is tell it like it was and hope you'll believe me that this was my life for real.

I wake to the sound of one hand clapping. It is my mother banging with the palm of her hand on the cellar door above me.

A moment before the air had been filled with the soft, heady scent of lavender. I was lying in a field, lilac-purple flowers swaying gently above me. The summer sun kissed my face, while giant white doves circled protectively in the clear, cloudless blue of the sky. I was safe. I was happy. I was, I thought, somewhere close to paradise.

Somewhere above me there is the sound of a wooden door creaking open. Then, the clunk of a light being switched on. I shut my eyes as a bright glare falls on me, a shaft of light piercing the empty darkness.

Slowly, I open them again. I'm blinded at first. The days spent imprisoned have got me used to the loneliness, the hunger and the dark. The giant white doves – my Loneliness Birds – are long gone. So are the Lavender Fields. My whole beautiful, magical world of make-believe has evaporated before my eyes.

Something scuttles across my feet, something slithering and animal. A mouse, perhaps. I pray not a rat. Where are my Loneliness Birds when I need them? As my eyes adjust to the harsh light, the bare brick walls of the cellar materialise all around me. My prison. I am in my prison. The prison of the nightmare of my childhood.

I glance down at my half-naked body. It is covered in livid red scratches and dark bluish bruises – the scars of my dirty, shameful, hate-filled existence. I shiver. It isn't from the cold. It's from the shame and the horror of the memories.

'Your father says it's time for you to come out of there.'

I hear the words from above. They are spoken in a tight, tense tone. The voice is familiar. It is my mother's. She'll never see me like this. She'll never come down those stairs, face to face with my naked abuse. For to do so would mean to acknowledge it, and she will choose today, as every day, the easy path, the path of wilful ignorance.

I sit upright, my aching back to the cold brick wall. I find my yellow trousers and shirt have been thrown in a heap next to me. I pull them on, wincing as I try to move my stiff, painful limbs. How long has it been this time? Two days? Three? Four?

Who knows?

Like so many times before, I have spent the lost days in my world of make-believe – my world of the Lavender Fields and the Loneliness Birds. For there I am warm and lovable and caressed and free, and it is there that I find my escape from the darkness.

'Hurry up!' Mum calls. 'Your father has visitors!'

I climb the stairs, forcing one painful limb before the other. I emerge from the dank cellar into the kitchen. Mum has already prepared a tray with tea and biscuits.

'Go tidy yourself up!' she scolds.

She can't bear to look at me. I am like a thing of dirt and guilt and shame, a dirty secret our family keeps hidden under the stairs. I feel such guilt. I want to say sorry. I want to tell my mother how much I love her and that I wish it would stop and that I am not making it happen. *It isn't me.* I'm sorry. I'm just a little child. I'm so guilty.

Instead, she orders me to the bathroom, to wash. There, I tie a scarf around my head, pushing all the greasy, matted strands away and underneath it. Then Mum shoves the tray of tea things into my hands and steers me out into the corridor, towards the men's room.

I walk the few steps to the front lounge as if in a daze, and knock on the door. Sitting on the floral pattern couches are several figures I recognise. All of them have long beards and traditional clothes – flowing jellabiya robes, and skullcaps. And at the centre of them all is their leader, the Imam of our mosque – my father.

At the sight of him I cast my eyes to the floor. Without a word, I go to set the tray down.

'Hello, it's Hannan!' says one of the men. 'Good to see her serving the guests. Good to see she's not being affected by these degenerate English ways, like a lot of young girls I could mention. How old is she now – seven?'

'Ah, no. Just turned six,' says Dad.

His gentle tone startles me, and I glance up at him. For one brief moment I look into his eyes. But there is nothing kind in them at all. Instead, they are filled with loathing and disgust.

I bow my head again, and back silently out of the room. Tears sting my eyes and begin to fall. I am, I know, somewhere close to hell.

I don't remember much from when I was little. The images are sketchy and opaque, a splash of colour here and there amongst the darkness and the dull smudge of grey. Maybe I have suppressed the memories. And who could blame me if I have?

But I do remember my street. My street was good fun. It was great on my street.

East Street, in Bermford, the north of England, was my playground. Two rows of identical, brick-built Victorian-era houses, with a leafy park at the top end. The trees were gnarled and twisty, and to me they seemed so huge. So tall and so old were they that I used to imagine they were monsters, complete with scary eyes and scary teeth. They cast their knotted, beast-like shadows over us while we played hide and seek amongst them, the tree-monsters adding a thrill of fear.

But I kept my ideas about the monster trees between my friends and myself. I would never tell my family. My family laughed at me so much about my daydreaming ways already.

It was normal for people to hang out on our street and pop into each other's houses. Doors were left open, and there was no fear of being robbed. I could wander down to my friend Amina's place whenever I felt like it. I was welcome to stay for as long as I wanted. If I was out for more than three or four hours, someone would come looking for me – my mother or one of my brothers. But it was still a kind of freedom for a little child.

I'd be offered a drink – squash or tea made in the traditional way. Water was boiled with tea leaves, and an equal amount of hot milk was added, plus lots of sugar and, sometimes, cardamom. And I'd be offered something to eat. It might be anything from chocolate digestives or Rich Tea biscuits, to curry and chapattis. It was typical of an Asian street in Britain in the early 1980s: a tight, close-knit community, where everyone knew each other.

My mother was a great cook, producing delicious, spicy meals on very little money. She would make chapattis using a special flour. She kneaded it with water to form a dough, then took a fist-sized blob, rolled it out into a flat circle on a chapatti iron, and cooked it until dark spots appeared on its surface. Or she'd make parathas, rolling out the dough into pancakes and placing them on a *tava* – a pan with a long handle. As she tossed them in the oil, they would puff up like little doughy balloons.

We would eat with our hands, using the chapatti or paratha as a scoop. Mum only ever used a knife to slice vegetables. She made her own samosas with spiced minced meat, or potato and peas. She made pakoras out of slices of onion and fresh chilli peppers, coated in a gram flour batter. She would drop these into a deep fryer filled with sizzling-hot oil. You knew when they were ready, for they would pop to the surface, all juicy golden brown.

My favourite dish was my mum's spicy okra curry – made with curry powder, garam masala, paprika, green chillies and tinned tomatoes. No one else could make it like she did. My favourite breakfast was 'eggy bread'. This is not a traditional food from Pakistan, as the rest of our meals generally were. But Mum liked it, and I simply adored it. She made eggy bread by soaking slices of white bread in raw egg, and frying them in oil. Scrumptious!

Across the way from our house were a Armenian family, a mother and her one son. This was one of the few families on our street who weren't of Pakistani Muslim origin. The Armenian lady used to try to communicate with Mum, but their English was very limited on both sides. Mum told us to call her 'Auntie', which is a traditional sign of respect. But Dad wouldn't have wanted us to. In private, he refused to show respect to anyone except other Pakistani Muslims. Even the Indian Muslims from around the corner weren't afforded true respect from him.

The Armenian 'Auntie' would bring over Armenian food for us. In return, Mum would take Pakistani delicacies to them. Luckily, Armenian Auntie was pretty good at remembering not to bring us pork. That wouldn't have gone down very well! Mostly, she cooked vegetarian hotpots – aubergines, potatoes and carrots stewed in a salty, peppery sauce. Before we were allowed to eat, Mum would go through the food with a fork, checking if there was any suspect meat. If there wasn't, we were free to tuck in.

Whenever the weather was good, our Armenian Auntie would bring a chair into her front yard. She'd sit there with her son, soaking up the rays and perhaps peeling some potatoes. We might stop to have a conversation if we were passing, but we would never go inside. She must have realised that for some reason she wasn't welcome in our home, and she didn't invite us into her house, either. Thankfully she wouldn't have known that the lack of welcome was due to my Dad hating white people.

A few doors down the street were a second Armenian family: a mother, a father, and a daughter. They were very different from Armenian Auntie. Whenever we saw them they would growl at us. They used to go to mass at an Orthodox Christian church, but the fact that they were Christians and we were Muslims didn't seem to be the issue. They would growl at anyone, regardless of their religion. I guess they were probably saying something in Armenian, but it didn't sound very nice. They just weren't 'people' people.

One or two of the rest of the houses on our street were rented out to students, so we'd often have different groups of young people living in them. One year, there were students from the Congo, in Central Africa. There were quite a lot of black Africans in my hometown, but they were the only ones on our street. And then there was the one house at the far end of the street with a lonely old white lady living in it.

Apart from that, everyone else on our street was a Muslim of Pakistani origin. In our part of town, there was only our street and one other that were like this – pretty much exclusively Pakistani Muslim territory. By the time I was a teenager, there would be even more Pakistani Muslims living there than when I was born.

The adults on my street dressed more or less as they would have done in the village in Pakistan. Women and men wore shalwar kamiz – a loose, matching smock top and trousers. The women's were more colourful, whilst the men had baggier trousers, in more sober, masculine colours – browns, greys and whites. Dad was always dressed in a white shalwar kamiz topped off with a *topi*, a traditional Punjabi skullcap.

Most of the men dressed like that except when they went to work. Work was generally in a Western environment and so they would wear Western clothes. They had a 'skin' that they would put on when they went out into the wider world. There, they had alternative identities as taxi drivers, policemen, engineers, and salespeople. But once back on the street they returned to life in the Pakistani village.

None of the women of my parents' generation worked, but some of the younger ones took jobs as secretaries or in shops, at least until they married. And when they went out to work, they too dressed in a more Western style. They still had to keep themselves properly covered, of course, and show appropriate modesty.

Four doors down from our house lived my Great-uncle Kramat and Great-auntie Sakina. They were like our surrogate grandparents, for our real ones were back in the village in Pakistan. But I didn't entirely like going to their house. I was scared of Uncle Kramat, who could be quite fierce with his big beard and bushy eyebrows. Both he and Auntie Sakina would gossip about my parents. They never really seemed to get along with my mum and dad, and I was never sure why.

Uncle Kramat and Auntie Sakina had three grown-up children – two sons, Ahmed and Saghir, and a daughter called Kumar. Ahmed was a bus driver. He owned the house rented to the African students, but he and his wife lived with Uncle Kramat and Auntie Sakina. His brother Saghir and his wife, plus Kumar and her husband, also lived there. So there were four married couples crammed into the one house, living as one big extended family. That wasn't so unusual on our street.

None of Uncle Kramat and Auntie Sakina's children had any offspring of their own. It seemed that they were unable to conceive. Some people on our street gossiped darkly that this was a punishment from Allah. Uncle Kramat was not a very religious man – or at least not 'religious' in the way that it was defined on our street. He had periods where he didn't go to the mosque. And he smoked *all* the time, which was seen as a very unholy thing to do.

Smoking wasn't around in the time of Mohammed, so the

Quran doesn't address it directly. But it does say: 'Do not with your own hands cast yourselves into destruction,' and, 'Do not kill yourselves'. Because smoking causes cancer, many pious Muslims interpret these verses as constituting a ban on smoking.

In our community good luck or bad luck would often be attributed to someone's moral or spiritual behaviour. Uncle Kramat's lack of piety was seen by all as the reason why his children were infertile. In all the gossiping on our street about why Uncle Kramat and Auntie Sakina had no grandchildren, no one ever mentioned the fact that Ahmed, Saghir and Kumar had married their first cousins – which is medically proven to increase the risk of being unable to conceive.

Uncle Kramat's children had tried in-vitro fertilisation. This was seen as yet a further transgression. If it was Allah's will that you didn't have children, then you were not supposed to interfere with that. You should just accept it.

Islam is first and foremost about submission to Allah's will. Indeed, a believer is often spoken of as 'the slave of God'. There is a common misconception that the primary meaning of Islam is 'peace', but this is true only in that a believer finds 'peace' by submitting to Allah's will.

My best friend on my street was Amina. She had unruly dark hair that fell to her shoulders in a wild tangle. I didn't think it was very pretty, and neither did she. But no one straightened their hair at the time, so she had to live with it. Amina's sister, Ruhama, was considered by far the prettier of the two. She had wavy hair that was more controllable. Both girls were paler-skinned than my sisters and me.

'She's so pretty!' people would remark of Ruhama. 'She's got such lovely hair, and such pale skin!'

When I overheard people saying this, I just presumed that dark skin was less beautiful somehow.

Amina's household seemed far more relaxed than mine. Her parents didn't pray regularly, and outside of her Quran lessons they rarely made her read the holy book. Neither she nor

Ruhama ever had to wear a hijab – the Muslim headscarf – when they were outside the house. They only ever wore one during Quran lessons at the mosque. But as my father was the community Imam, I had to wear one at all times.

Amina, Ruhama and I were forever playing hopscotch. We'd get chalk and draw a course on the pavement. The paving stones formed squares, so we just had to write the numbers inside each. The rules were dead simple: throw a stone and hop onto the single square, then jump with both feet onto the double square. If your feet touched any of the lines – or cracks in the pavement in our case – then you were out. The next person would take their go, and try to get further than you.

We started timing each other – counting from one to one hundred, and seeing who could do it the fastest. Ruhama was great, but I wasn't so agile or so focussed. Halfway through I would lose my attention and start daydreaming. My world wasn't always happy, and the only escape I had was to make up another one.

My favourite place was either in my room or at Amina's house. My favourite pastime was reading. I spent a lot of my waking hours reading, making up stories, and drawing pictures. Most of my doodles showed a little cottage with a pretty flower garden. This was my fantasy home. In reality we had a tiny back yard, where Mum grew mint and coriander. There were no flowers: Mum had no time or space for growing them.

My favourite time of year was the fifth of November, when Bonfire Night took over our street. For days on end everyone would join forces building up a huge bonfire from waste wood, fallen branches and old packing crates. Each household would buy whatever fireworks and sparklers they could afford. November was always cold, but we'd wrap up warm in woolly scarves and hats. Then we'd gather excitedly for the fire to be lit. I loved that moment – the wonderful, tingling anticipation of it all going up in a big whoosh of flames.

Normally, the men of the street would douse the bonfire in some old sump oil. Then they'd warn us all to stand back, and set it alight. All of a sudden it would go up in a big whump, throwing a burning heat across our faces and with sparks flying high into the dark sky. Soon we'd be roasting potatoes and marshmallows over the flames, and warming our hands and faces, and munching 'bonfire' – treacle – toffee.

The Armenian family from across the street would be there, as were the African students who lodged in my uncle's house. It was the one time of year when everyone on our street was truly united – all except for my father. He would stand outside our house with a disapproving air about him. Dad hated seeing people having fun.

Because Christmas and Easter were overtly Christian affairs, the community wasn't allowed to do anything to celebrate then. But Dad didn't really know what Bonfire Night was about, because he knew nothing about the traditions or history of England, the country he had made his home. My dad believed that England was a land of immorality, populated by infidels, and he only cared to know about the land and religion of his birth.

In my father's eyes, Bonfire Night was wholly a white English affair, and not for us. But he couldn't think of any 'religious' justification for banning it. Everyone enjoyed it so much, and he would have had a real fight on his hands if he had tried to put a stop to it. Instead, he made sure that he never joined in, and that everyone knew he disapproved.

At the bottom of our street was a parallel road leading up to West Albion Street. There was little or no reason to go that way, because school and the town centre lay in the other direction. There were several posh houses there, with big gardens and iron gates. Gleaming Land Rovers and Mercedes were parked in the driveways, and the owners had fierce, Rottweiler-type dogs. The kids in those houses would play with each other, and we stayed away because of the dogs. They lived a completely separate life from us, and we knew we'd never end up playing in their gardens.

Up the other end of the street was 'Jack' the Jack Russell's house. Though he was a lot smaller than the Rottweilers, he was no less vicious. This tiny ball of fluff would go racing out of his owner's house if he spotted any of us passing, growling and yapping as he ran. If he caught you, his bite was just as bad as his bark!

One day two of my friends were coming home from town. They turned into our street and Jack spotted them. 'Jack! Jack!' his owner cried. 'Come back here!' But Jack could not be stopped. My friends were running towards their house as fast as their legs would carry them, but one, Saira, was too slow. Jack caught Saira and sank his teeth into her leg.

As soon as we heard what had happened Mum and I went round to visit. Gingerly, Saira took the bandage off to show us the damage. There were puncture marks where Jack's teeth had gone in, and stitches all around the wound. It was certainly dramatic, and I was very impressed. Saira had had to have a tetanus jab in her bottom, in case Jack had poisoned her.

Saira's parents were angry. There was a Pakistani Muslim who lived on a neighbouring street and he was a policeman. Anyone with a serious problem on our street always took it to him, and Saira's parents reported Jack for biting their daughter. He insisted on filing a police report, and he told Jack's owner that the dog would have to be muzzled. But Jack never was.

Jack's owner was a little old white woman, and the last white British person living on our street. Sometimes, when it was sunny, she'd sit on a chair outside her door. But we never said hello to her, because we were too scared of Jack. In any case, she had her own visitors from within her community, and their lives never really touched ours.

Opposite Jack's place was a run-down house set on its own among thick bushes. It looked dark and mysterious, and my brothers used to say that the Bogeyman lived there. I believed them, and I hated walking past. I thought of the Bogeyman as a monster with some horrible disfigurement on his face – what else could explain why he stayed inside all the time? And I imagined that he was a white person, because someone had once said: *I saw the Bogeyman; he's white like a ghost.* We told each other frightening stories of what the Bogeyman would do if he caught us. Zakir, the oldest of my brothers, said that the Bogeyman ate children for breakfast.

With the park and its monster trees, and Jack the vicious Jack Russell, and the Bogeyman, this really was the scary end of the street. As soon as I approached it I would start running, and I wouldn't stop until I was down the 'safe' end of the street.

But in reality I was far from safe. I was never safe, because my father was the real Bogeyman.

Chapter Two

To Pakistan, with Love

My parents came from a very rural existence and a farming background. Yet in Britain my mum and dad lived a totally urban life, blocked in the whole time by brick walls and tarmac. Months would go by with their lives confined almost entirely to the interior of the house, our street and the nearby mosque.

My mother loved to go outdoors, but she had six children and a husband to look after. She had to do all the washing, ironing, cooking and cleaning for a household of eight, and that took up most of her time. She wouldn't have been able to survive such a life without her uncles, aunts and relatives around her. She needed them, just like she needed the nearby shops that sold the traditional ingredients that she liked: halal meat, spices, okra and chapatti flour. In effect, my parents had recreated their Pakistani village existence in East Street. If anything, because it covered only the one street, our community was even more restricted than the village had been.

Going back a generation, my granddad wouldn't have been able to cope with life in the city. If ever he went to Islamabad, or any big town in Pakistan, he would want to get out again right away. But my parents were running from rural Pakistan: it was a poverty trap from which they had escaped by emigrating. An English town had running water, electricity, free education and shops crammed full of every good imaginable. They had none of this back in the villages from where they came. There, toilets were nothing more than long drop holes in the ground. And as for schooling, education opportunities for rural villagers were basically non-existent.

Growing up in a rural Pakistani village, my father had finished his education at age eleven. From then on he went to the madrassa, a religious school that teaches the Quran, and nothing but the Quran. My mother was even less well educated. After just one year of village schooling she was barely able to read or write. We spoke Punjabi or, occasionally, Urdu – but never English – at home.

My father was in his late twenties when he came to the United Kingdom. He had been a farmer in the Punjab, an area on the border between India and Pakistan. In religious terms he was a Deobandi Sunni Muslim, a strand of Islam found across much of the tribal areas of northern India, Pakistan and Afghanistan.

When he first came to the UK Dad lived in a rented house in a town in Lancashire, with lots of other Pakistani men from the same tribal area. Fifteen or twenty of them were piled in together in one terraced house. Dad spoke no English, and neither did the others. They had little need of it, either at home or at work.

The men came over to work in the textile factories. As soon as they could, they helped each other to buy houses. They hardly ever spent money on anything other than food, and housing. Dad and my friend Skip's father saved up their earnings year on year, and bought a house together in my home town. Mortgages weren't part of the culture back in the village in Pakistan, so they bought it outright. Two years or so after buying that house their wives came over to join them.

Mum and Dad had married before he left to go to England. It was an arranged marriage, according to tradition. She came from a nearby village in an equally impoverished rural area. The opportunity to move abroad and to better your life was something that most people would jump at. Gradually, the street that Mum and Dad moved into was taken over by Pakistani families, and the white English people moved out.

My father didn't like non-Muslims. This was the sixties and seventies – a time of flower power, drugs and free love, of men wearing 'weird clothes' and growing their hair long. My parents didn't approve of any of this, and they didn't like the 'disrespectful' way that English children spoke to their parents. They didn't like what they saw as the lack of English 'community spirit', and so they created their own, Pakistani Muslim, community on our street. They were determined not to allow English culture to spill over into our street and 'pollute' their community.

At home, Dad was a distant figure. He would spend his time cloistered with his holy book. He would be continually murmuring verses of the Quran, while fingering his *tasbih* – his prayer beads. The tasbih looks almost exactly like Catholic rosary beads. Some are made of wood, some of marble. There are ninety-nine beads altogether, and they are arranged with four exactly the same, and then one slightly larger – so you can work your way around the beads by touch alone.

Dad would always have his tasbih in his hand, even if he was walking down the street. He had little tasbihs sent over from Pakistan, for my brothers and me. By the age of four he'd taught me to flick the beads through my fingers while reciting the ninety-nine names of Allah. Chanting these names – *Irahma*, the Gracious; *Rahim*, the Merciful; *Malik*, the Sovereign – is supposed to bring you a deeper sense of holiness.

But to me these were just foreign words, ones that I didn't even understand. As with Quran chanting, Dad taught me how to say them – not what they meant. I was just ordered to do it. I learnt these mysterious words to try to please him. But when I did manage to learn all ninety-nine off by heart, he didn't even reward me with a smile, or a 'well done'. He just wheeled me out in front of guests and made me perform the tasbih. The more he didn't show me any appreciation, the more I felt a desperate hunger to try to do something to earn his blessing.

Dad's existence revolved around his idea of how a man should lead a religious life. His main concerns were praying five times a day, and going to the mosque to preach. Quite often, he would travel to Lancaster, Manchester or Birmingham, if there were religious events at mosques there. He had no hobbies outside his religious life, except for watching television. Even then it was preferably a video of a holy man giving a lesson, or some qawwali music – a style of Sunni singing popular in Pakistan. His 'social life' was limited to talking with his male friends, usually in the men's lounge in our house.

There were halal restaurants in our area, but my parents never went to them. Going out for a meal wasn't part of their culture. In any case, my father wouldn't trust them to give him real halal food. A lot of the men in our community led similar lives to Dad's: very simple, very frugal, and very much closed off from the world around them.

Dad was not a practical man. My brothers and Mum did all the decorating and odd jobs around the house. If a bulb was gone or a light fitting was loose, my dad would order my brothers to fix it. If it was beyond my brothers' abilities, he would ring up Uncle Ahmed. By virtue of being the Imam, Dad was seen to exist on a higher spiritual plane. Such worldly things as fixing a radiator were beneath him. There was far more 'honour' in being an Imam than being a bus driver or a handyman – so Ahmed felt he owed my dad. Dad did more to 'honour' Ahmed by being his Imam than Ahmed did to Dad by doing DIY jobs around the home.

Each year my parents would try to make a visit to Pakistan. When I was three years old they took me with them, leaving my brothers in the care of some relatives on our street. At that time none of my sisters had yet been born. We travelled to Pindi Khan, a tiny, mud-walled village in the Punjab, sandwiched between the North-West Frontier Province and Kashmir.

This was my father's home village. It was the rainy season, and I remember it being surrounded by green fields, and with a river running through it. In the dry season it would get parched and desert-like, the fields turning into brown patches of sandy dust. Pindi Khan is in a very rural and isolated area. Everyone living there is related, and all are part of the one tribe. Cousins, distant cousins, and second cousins twice removed – people would only marry within their clan lines. That was the tradition. Inter-marriage was part of the defence system of clans that seemed to be permanently at war.

17

Life in Pindi Khan was simple. People would earn a little money from selling wheat, milk, cattle, goats and eggs. Animals rather than machinery were used to plough, reap and sow. We travelled around on a *tonga*, a traditional horse and cart. The local boys would be educated either at the madrassa, or at the village school, but few girls would get any education. The madrassa was better funded, and seen as providing a better education. In the villages, next to nothing was invested in public schooling. The madrassa would be run by a local Imam, and supported by donations.

My dad kept a house in the village. It was brick-built, with several rooms arranged around a central courtyard. Each room was flat-roofed, so you could sit out and even sleep on the roof if you wanted to. To begin with, Dad had nurtured an ambition to return to live in the village. Over the years, he had kept adding to that house. Eventually, when it became clear we weren't going to return, it became more of a home for us when visiting.

Shortly after our arrival in Pindi Khan we were sitting out in the courtyard. My parents were having morning tea. The gate was open, and in the field in front of the house was a clothesline. I wandered out of the gate and disappeared under the clothesline. A little while later Mum realised that she had lost sight of me. She went out to look. There was I in the middle of the field, sitting under an enormous cow. This was one of the family herd, which were kept mainly for milk.

The cow seemed to be standing guard over me, as if I was her calf. Mum called one of Dad's sisters and pointed, and together they burst out laughing. But at the same time they were worried that the cow might step on me. They rushed over and whisked me up, to save me from being trampled.

A few days later we were sitting in the field, with the goats grazing all around us. I was playing with some coins in the grass. A goat nuzzled up to me and I offered it a coin. Goats eat anything, and this one licked the coin straight out of my hand and swallowed it. The coin was a paisa, worth less than a penny. Mum thought it was simply hilarious. She told everyone in the village. Partly the joke was that I was so unused to rural Punjabi life that I fed money to a goat. And partly, it was that the goat had actually eaten the coin.

When we got back to the UK Mum seemed very proud that she had taken her eldest daughter 'home'. She was forever telling visitors about it.

'Hannan went to the village, you know. She seemed so at home there in Pakistan, a good Muslim country. She was adopted by a cow and even fed a paisa to a goat!'

When she wasn't crushed down under her burden of work, Mum had a great sense of humour. But I wondered if I had really felt 'at home' in Pakistan. I couldn't remember exactly. My concept of what the village was like came from my own hazy memories, and from my mother's stories of what life had been like 'back home' in her day.

Mum was forever reminiscing with her friends. She painted life in the village as being quite magical: neighbours sharing houses and supporting each other, and helping in the fields with the crops, and cooking curry and chapattis for each other. Mum loved telling the story of how she had left the village and come to the North of England, and her words had a wistful tone whenever she did. Mum and her friends on the street seemed to share a romanticised vision of village life, where everyone was one big happy family.

Letters from aunts, uncles and cousins would be passed around. It was from these that we got a more realistic sense of the way of life and the culture in Pakistan. We would learn of uncles who had gone to places like Dubai or Saudi Arabia seeking work, for there were no opportunities in the village. After six months they would return enriched by their savings, as 'big men' in the village. Or we would hear news of births, marriages and deaths in our extended family. But most of this meant very little to me. I didn't know who these people were, so why should I care?

My parents wanted us to learn all about Pakistan, the 'home country'. We were supposed to read books in Urdu about the post-colonial partition of India that created Pakistan. We were supposed to read about the life of Mohammed Ali Jinnah, the man who oversaw partition and became the first Governor-General. But my sole experience of Pakistan was one short visit when I was three years old. I lived in England, and it was England that felt like the 'home country' to me.

Whenever we had news from Pakistan, my brothers would mutter: 'God! We're so glad we don't live there!'

They were careful to do so in English, so my parents couldn't understand. They were my sentiments exactly! My brothers valued their lives in Britain because it was a land of opportunity, when compared to rural Pakistan. Britain had simple luxuries like running water, electricity and tarmac roads. But it was also because they knew the restrictions they would be living under in Pakistan.

They loved watching football on TV and hanging out with their schoolmates, wearing Western clothes and listening to pop bands. In Pakistan they would have none of this. They would spend their time at a madrassa – a religious school – learning to memorise the Quran, praying at the mosque, and working on the farm. We had plenty of cousins back in the village who led exactly that life, and it was one that none of us wanted to emulate.

But there were people on our street who seemed to pine for that sort of existence. We used to call them 'Pakis'. We used the word 'Paki' a lot, and to us it signified someone who was wedded to the old ways. When my sister Sabina came along, she would prove to be a real 'Paki' herself in that sense. After Mum and Dad took her back to the village, she never stopped talking about it.

'Oh, I loved it there,' Sabina would tell us. 'Everyone is so religious.'

Pakistan has this. Pakistan has that. We used to tire of listening to her. Sometimes we'd call her a real 'Paki' to her face. She seemed almost proud of it. Of course, if an outsider had called any of us a 'Paki', there would be racist undertones that we'd react against. We knew that the word 'Paki' could be used as a racist taunt. Each of us would have it thrown at us at one time or another in our lives.

We also had a term we used for a white person – *gora*. This wasn't insulting – it just means 'white person'. As with the term Paki, it depended upon who used it and how it was used. In my father's mouth *gora* was a racist insult. He made no bones about the fact that he abhorred white people and their ways. He spent his time at home, or at the mosque, and he only ever ran into *gora* when he couldn't avoid it.

I used to see the odd news story on the TV about Pakistan. It always seemed to be so dusty and dry. In parts it was practically a baking hot desert. It was tough to make a living from farming, but for most that was the only way to survive. The wealth and status of a man was generally measured in how many livestock he owned.

Recently, however, a new form of status had entered into the equation – how many family members one might have living overseas, in the UK, the USA or across Europe. This was part of the contradictory view of the West that permeated Pakistani rural society. On the one hand, everything Western was hateful; on the other, it was a sign of real achievement having family living and working there.

Having family abroad was far more important in terms of wealth and status than if one had been on the Hajj – the pilgrimage to Mecca, the site of Islam's holiest shrines. Of course, the Hajj was supposed to be the real measure of a person's worth – but having livestock and family abroad were the things that really mattered.

'Ali has done really well,' so-and-so would remark. 'His son has been to the UK, and got a job and married there.'

Whatever job someone had secured overseas – even if it was packing pizzas into boxes – he would still be able to earn enough to return to Pakistan as a 'big man'. The money in his pocket would be so much more than anyone else would have. Not surprisingly, whenever Mum and Dad went back to the village they were treated like celebrities. Emigration is one of the few routes out of the grinding poverty of rural life that otherwise continues unchanged from generation to generation.

As with many in immigrant communities, people like my

parents left Pakistan for Britain seeing it as a temporary sojourn. The plan was to earn some money and return home. But as time went by most decided to bring their wives and families over, and settle down. And yet so many of the people on our street resented British culture, and tried to isolate themselves from it completely.

It hadn't taken my father long to realise that the British education system was vastly superior to anything available in rural Pakistan. He knew by staying in Britain his family would have access to it. And that would give his sons a much better chance of success in life. That is what he stayed for. He didn't care about his daughters' education. They were only good for marrying off and having children. But he wanted his sons to do well.

I was the fourth child born to my parents, and the first girl. At first, my brothers were so happy to have a little sister. Zakir was my eldest brother, and he was Mum's favourite. He would stick up for me in school or in the street if he saw anyone being nasty to me. But in the privacy of our home my father and brothers were allowed to be nasty to me – for I was 'only a girl'.

Zakir was also a know-it-all that everyone described as the 'brains' of the family. He was football crazy, and obsessed with football stickers and magazines. He'd do 'swapsies' with his friends, and somehow always managed to get exactly what he wanted. He was so jammy. But most of all I resented him because he got on so well with Mum and Dad.

The next brother was Raz, and he was the most religious of the boys. He wasn't radical, just spiritual. From an early age the mosque was his life. He didn't do well at school, and he wasn't bothered about studying mainstream subjects. His main interest lay in the Quran, and his second great love was football.

My third and favourite brother was Billy. Billy was actually his nickname – it means 'cat' in Punjabi. He'd got that name because he was slinky and feline – like a cat. He was also gentle, considerate, and charming. With his dark, rakish good looks, all the girls would fancy him when he grew up. Billy tried to help in the house, but my father would always stop him. That wasn't the 'right' sort of work for boys.

Billy was my favourite because he was the only one who was ever vaguely nice to me. Billy was also the family peacemaker. We were forever fighting over what to watch on TV. Billy would try to talk everyone into taking it in turns.

After me, there were two more girls. The first was Sabina. Like Raz, she was very religious, though her faith was far more conservative. Sabina grew up with an active dislike of English culture. She didn't like going to school. She didn't like mixing with boys. She had few or no white friends. With her natural affinity for traditional Pakistani culture, she was the perfect daughter for Mum and Dad that I never was.

After Sabina there was a gap of a few years, and then Mum had Aliya. Aliya was very pretty and dainty, and she was Dad's favourite out of the girls. He was actually quite soft with her. She would go and sit on his lap, and fire questions at him: *if you pray like this, what will happen?* To my amazement, he would see fit to answer her.

In our culture girls are less welcome than boys. We are presumed to be in need of constant protection. This wasn't just for our own good; it was for the sake of the family's honour. If a daughter goes off the rails, it brings more shame on your family than if a son does. I never heard any of the women on the street gossiping about boys doing anything wrong. It just wasn't a big deal. The gossip was always about the girls.

The culture on our street was very much centred around how you could gain honour, how you could maintain that honour, and how you could avoid bringing shame on yourself or your family. The women were obsessed with honour and shame. It was by listening to their gossip that we learned what was appropriate and what was not, and how an individual family's honour and shame were computed.

By the time that I was born Dad had left his factory job and started working as the local Imam – the community's spiritual leader. He didn't earn a wage as such. Instead, he survived on benefits, and on what the community donated.

We didn't have many luxuries at home. Most of the family's

clothes came from charity shops. Before my sisters came along I shared a bedroom with Mum, and then all we females shared the one room together, sometimes sharing beds too. Like many Pakistani couples, my parents never slept in the same room. Dad slept in the front lounge. My oldest brother, Zakir, had his own room, and the other boys shared.

My sisters and I wore traditional shalwar kamiz – a long smock top and matching trousers – always. These were made by Mum on a Singer electric sewing machine. She would work on the clothes in the kitchen when we were at school. Other women on the street might pay her a little to make outfits for weddings or festivals. If money was tight, Mum would put the money so earned towards the family food budget. If it wasn't, she might buy us a treat. One thing she would never do was spend it on herself.

Mum really enjoyed making clothes, and she was at her happiest when doing so. She would get excited about a new project, and be proud of the end result. There was only one problem: she always insisted on dressing me in garish bright yellow. She said it looked nice on me, but I hated it. I didn't tell her as much. I didn't think she would listen.

Shortly after the visit to the village, we acquired a fat cat with dark brown fur. She was our first ever pet. We immediately gave her the name 'Billy' – 'cat' in Punjabi! So now we had Billy my brother and Billy the cat. My brothers and I loved to play with her. I'd get her to crawl all over them while chasing after a ball of string. But Dad just ignored her. He didn't like her being around, especially when he was reading the Quran. Cats were dirty creatures, he said, and Billy had to be left outside.

One day Billy was whining and she looked to be in pain. She also seemed to be very fat. I asked mum what was wrong with her.

'Oh, it's nothing,' Mum replied. 'Just she might be about to have babies.'

I was amazed. I thought we'd been overfeeding her. Mum brought Billy's basket into the kitchen, and for the next few days we fed her warm milk. Early one morning she gave birth to eight kittens. But within hours four of them had died. It was so sad. Mum told us that we had to choose one to keep from the survivors. That really got me and my brothers going.

'Let's have this one!'

'No, this is the nicest!'

'This one! This one! It's just opened its eyes!'

Once we'd chosen our one, we had to find homes for the other three. Funnily enough we decided to call our second cat 'Billy' as well. So now we had 'Billy One' and 'Billy Two' – plus the original Billy, my brother. But soon after she'd given birth Billy One started to get very aggressive – first towards Billy Two, and then towards us. She was scratching and going wild.

Eventually, without breathing a word to me, my brothers decided to get rid of Billy One. They took her in a car somewhere far away and abandoned her. I missed Billy One when she was gone but no one ever told me what had happened to her. And no one ever explained how Billy One had become pregnant. I didn't dare ask. Such questions didn't usually go down very well in my household.

From my earliest years I was steeped in my family's religion, Islam. It dominated our lives from dawn to dusk. My father taught me about the Five Pillars of Islam, the foundations of our faith. Anyone who adhered to the Five Pillars was on the path to Paradise, he said. The Five Pillars are one, the declaration of faith; two, giving money to the poor; three, fasting during the holy month of Ramadan; four, Hajj, the pilgrimage to Mecca; and five, praying five times a day.

From the age of three my biggest daily task was learning the Quran. It is seen as being honourable for a Muslim to have learned to read the Quran. It brings shame on the family if you reach a certain age without having done so. There was a man on our street who was infamous, for he had never learned to read Arabic. This meant he couldn't read or recite any of the Quran, for it has to be both learnt and spoken in classical Arabic, the original language in which it was written.

Not only did I have to learn the Quran, I had to do so in a language I neither understood nor spoke – Arabic. My parents' native tongues are Urdu and Punjabi, and we usually spoke Punjabi at home. My dad ran formal Quran lessons for all the children on our street below the age of five. Five days a week we would crowd into the guest room at the front of the house, a room that doubled as my dad's bedroom. Woebetide any of us who got my father's lessons wrong.

On one wall of the lounge was a picture of the Kaaba, the holiest place in Islam. The Kaaba is a cube-like building situated in Mecca, Saudi Arabia, the Muslim Holy Land. It stands about fifteen metres high and ten or twelve wide, and is draped in the kiswah, a black silk cloth embroidered with Quranic verses. It is a simple structure made of granite, and it is said to have been built by Abraham and Ishmael.

Dad told us that the Kaaba is venerated because it contains the first ever Quran, upon which the Prophet Mohammed recorded the holy word of God. In fact, he had it completely wrong. The Kaaba is empty, apart from a meteorite called the Black Stone embedded in the southeast corner. This was just one example of my father's lack of knowledge of his faith – of Islam. But of course, as an infant child I had no way of realising his ignorance, or of challenging it.

On the opposite wall of our lounge was a framed saying in raised gold lettering: 'Mohammed, peace be upon him'. It was in Arabic, of course. Below that was a cabinet containing crockery that was only ever used on special occasions, and two glass snowstorms. One was a snowstorm over the Kaaba, the other a storm of snowflakes swirling around the name of the Prophet Mohammed. We never got them out and played with them. To have done so would have been 'disrespectful'. It would have attracted my father's wrath, and that, I knew, was best avoided.

On the top shelf of the cabinet were a number of Qurans. It is respectful to keep the holy book in a high place. Each was covered in a tiny cloth sleeve made by Mum from odd bits of material left over from her sewing. There were two settees in the lounge that could be converted into beds. During Quran lessons, they would be pushed to one side, and a rug would be put down for us Quran students to sit on.

We sat in a square of twelve, facing inwards, with Dad at the head. Each of us had a wooden *rail* – a bookstand – with an Arabic dictionary, or a verse of the Quran, propped on it. Boys and girls sat together, and we didn't have to wear uniform or anything. But these classes were still joyless affairs. One by one, we'd each sit by Dad, and recite the day's lesson. The serious atmosphere in the room contrasted with the bright, 1970s floral patterns on the wallpaper, carpet and even the settees.

Dad was very strict. No one ever misbehaved. The most one of the kids would ever do was whisper to a friend, and even that resulted in a sharp whack. Dad had a broom handle that he kept in one corner. He didn't need to wield it very often: the very presence of it by his side was enough to keep order. If we didn't recite the Arabic perfectly, we knew we'd be beaten. We were told that the words had a particular spiritual significance in Arabic, which was lost if spoken in any other language. That's why we couldn't do the lessons in English, a language we all understood.

We were never taught the actual meaning of the words we recited – just the pitch-perfect Arabic pronunciation. I might recognise proper names, like 'Allah' and 'Mohammed'. Beyond that, I didn't have a clue what any of it meant. But none of us ever questioned anything, or sought meaning or asked for explanations. I wouldn't have dreamt of asking my father a single question. I was too scared of him.

At first, we learned the classical Arabic alphabet. Arabic is written from right to left, and the words are joined up with few spaces. Then we moved on to learning the verses. But Dad couldn't show us how to write it, because writing down the words of the Quran is 'disrespectful'. We were simply given the first ayah – or verse – and had to stare at it and try to figure out the Arabic letters and words. We had to say the same sentence over and over, maybe for an hour or more, until Dad judged that we had it right. Then we could move on to the next one.

I learned to read that first Surah pitch-perfect when I was just five years old. I was one of the first in the class to do so. Dad was forever encouraging the other girls and boys, but he never seemed to say a word of praise to me. I had learned that Surah off by heart to try to please him. But he never so much as smiled, or acknowledged my achievement for one instant.

In a way, I wasn't particularly surprised. Dad had made no bones about the fact that he never wanted a daughter. In private, he told me that I was an evil, cursed girl. He said that it was up to me to prove to him that I wasn't bad and useless and stupid, and 'unworthy of Allah'.

Because my father was the Imam, my parents were seen as pillars of the community. My father had an exalted status on our street. To outsiders he appeared as sweet and gentle as can be. He spoke almost in a whisper, smiled a lot, and seemed so friendly. He acted like a truly spiritual and peaceable person. He was especially like that with people from outside the community. That's what people saw.

'What a lovely father you have,' they'd tell me.

Little did they know. Even at four years old, I knew Dad wasn't lovely at all. In private, he was full of cruel words and hatred, of rage and violence. Often, he lashed out physically at Mum. I didn't have to be told that this was wrong. My instincts said that it was. But even though I knew he wasn't perfect, like any child I still wanted my father to love and be proud of me – hence my efforts to succeed at my Quran studies. It was just a pity that all that innocent effort and hope was so wasted.

People from the community called my father 'Hajji', meaning one who has been on the pilgrimage to Mecca. They addressed my mother by the feminine form, 'Hajjin'. They described Dad as being 'humble'. If you asked anyone in our community what they meant by 'humility', they would say that it was someone who prayed a lot and read the Quran. In that sense Dad was 'humble'. People saw him as their source of guidance and wisdom, and they would come to seek his advice.

People would ask my father: *should we tell our daughter to behave in this or that way?* Dad would always give a response. With my father, uncertainty or ambivalence were unheard of. He always acted as if he knew exactly how to advise people, often peppering his advice with references to 'holy scriptures'.

Whenever people came to ask his advice, it would impress on me that my father was somehow special. It also increased the pressure on me not to do anything that might be seen as bad. Other mothers looked upon me as a role model. They scrutinised my behaviour much more closely. If I did something 'shameful', then it would reflect upon the whole community, for my father was their holy man.

Having a daughter who misbehaved would have been the ultimate dishonour for my father. And it would have been bad news for the street as a whole.

So I never stood a chance really – for I was a born rebel.

Chapter Three

Jane and Susan

My life and that of my brothers was an exercise in reading between the lines. Rules were rarely specified. I had to work out what was allowed, and what was not, by listening to the gossip. Even having a white person visit your house would be the subject for gossip. And we had all heard Dad express his views on white people, and their decadent culture.

Dad was forever ranting about 'goray' – white people. According to Dad, a gora was a 'Godless, heathen fornicator'. They drank alcohol and were sexually loose. You only had to look at the clothes they wore to know this. Women freely showing off flesh – arms, legs and even cleavage! – to tempt men. My father wanted none of his offspring to have anything to do with gora-kind.

On our street my brothers hung out with other Pakistani Muslim boys. But they did have white friends at school. Whenever Dad wasn't around they would talk about friends with exotic names like 'Tim', 'Andy' and 'Peter'. But they never tried to bring their gora friends home. They knew Dad would refuse them entry to the house. Once, Zakir did walk back from school with his white friend, Dave. But he found an excuse to make Dave wait for him outside the front gate.

The rule against white people was entirely my father's. His fear was two-fold. He believed it was his religious duty to reject foreigners. The Quran does warn believers not to take Jews and Christians for their friends, although in other places it includes altogether more positive comments about them. And my father's fear was cultural: he worried that English ways would somehow 'infect' his family, and lead us off the straight and narrow.

As for Mum, she didn't seem to share such fears at all. But it was my father's will that ruled in our house, and she had to do as he said. She knew very well that none of us were allowed to have white visitors, even as little children.

When I was four years old I started going to nursery school. There I made friends with two sisters, Jane and Susan. Mum and I would often walk most of the way home with them, as their street was two away from ours. Mum was forever smiling and laughing and being playful with them. Sometimes, she would bring me a treat: biscuits or crisps or some toffee sweets. She'd make sure I shared them with Jane and Susan, regardless of the fact that they were white.

But it was all very different at home. It was fine for Jane and Susan to play with me in the back yard. But they had to be kept out of the house. And if Dad was around, they weren't welcome in the back yard even. For poor Mum it was a delicate balancing act. She didn't want to be unwelcoming to my friends. She'd bring us our biscuits and squash in the yard, and try to make us feel at home. But growing up in Pakistan she'd been taught never to question her husband or defy his will – doubly so if he was also the community Imam.

Jane was nearer to me in age and she was my best friend. Girls make and break friends quite a lot at that age, but we were close for a long time. She was very self-confident, not introverted like me. Her sister, Susan, had dramatic, flowing red hair, but Jane's was straight and brown. The other girls teased her by calling her 'Plain Jane'. But I thought her hair far finer than my thick, unruly black locks. Jane never let the teasing get to her. She gave as good as she got.

Jane and I sat next to each other at nursery. She loved the sound of her own voice, and could rabbit on and on. As for me, I was a follower, not a leader. I was very loyal, and I could listen and listen. We were a perfect match. At four years old my days at the nursery with Jane were my escape from the suffocating nature of life at home. With a best friend like her I could have been so happy, if not for my father.

*

My dad was erratic and unpredictable when it came to many things, but especially his food. He used meals as an excuse to attack Mum, both verbally and physically. The first time I remember this happening was when I was four.

Mum was serving Dad some curry in the back lounge. The front room was reserved for receiving guests, and was really only for the men to use. The back lounge was where we gathered to watch TV – the only truly communal activity we ever did as a family. We never spoke much, so we didn't gather there to chat.

My mother handed my father his plate of curry. I saw him scoop up a handful with a chunk of chapatti, but just as soon as he put it in his mouth his face turned dark as thunder.

'This isn't cooked properly,' he snapped. 'It's cold! You stupid woman! I can't eat this!'

With that, he hurled the food at the wall. The plate smashed upon impact, brown slugs of food dribbling down the wallpaper. Dad got to his feet, and started yelling at Mum. She backed away from him in terror, but it only made things worse. He began screaming at her for trying to get away when he was talking. She was pleading with him to calm down, but he went storming after her into the kitchen.

I was left alone in the lounge. From there I could hear the dull thump of his fist smashing into her body, as Mum screamed and screamed. He beat her again and again and again and again. I could hear every blow. I sat there frozen to the spot, with tears streaming down my face. I was crying from fear. I was so scared for Mum. I feared that he might kill her.

Dad had never raised a hand to me before now, so my fear was all for Mum. She pleaded with him to stop, but the merciless pounding continued. My mum's screams were so loud that I was sure the neighbours would hear. But Dad was the community Imam, and by definition a holy man. Even if they did hear the beating, they would never challenge or question him, let alone interfere.

Finally he stormed out of the kitchen and into his domain –

the front lounge. I crept out to the kitchen, which was at the back of the house. I wanted to comfort Mum, and I wanted her to comfort me. I found her curled into a foetal position lying on the floor. I reached out to help her, but she wouldn't let me touch, and she pushed me away. Mum was ashamed for her little, four-year-old daughter to see her like this.

When Mum finally managed to get to her feet she could barely walk. But she knew it was her job to clear up the mess. She had to kneel on her painful knees to pick up the pieces of broken plate, and put them into the dustpan, along with the congealed lumps of curry. Then she had to sponge the sticky mess out of the carpet, so as not to leave a stain. Later, Dad emerged from his room seemingly as if nothing had happened.

I was soon to realise that this was the pattern of his violent behaviour. Every time he beat Mum up, things just went on as normal. She cleared up the mess, whilst trying to hide her hurt and her wounds from us all, and the neighbours, and Dad acted as if nothing had happened. This was one of the things that made me so angry: by silently taking the beatings, Mum was trying to protect my father, the family, and our 'honour'.

I realised that Dad was beating up Mum this badly once a month or so. The reason could be anything: 'bad' cooking; the tea not as he wanted it; clothes washed and ironed 'improperly'; the house not perfectly clean to receive his guests. I was starting to realise that things were rotten somewhere in Dad's relationship with us.

But a child always lives in hope. I lived in the hope that things would get better, and that Dad would be the loving and caring father that I dreamed him to be. He would stop beating Mum. He would notice me, and show me just a little love and affection. He would praise me, just the once, for my Quran recitals. And all in my life would be good.

Faced with an abuser, it is easy to believe that all you have to do is be good enough for them, and they will stop. Sadly, the reverse is so much more often true.

*

I started junior school aged five. I was very shy and hardly ever spoke in class. The teachers thought I was a nice, kind person, but that I was far too shy and quiet. The same was true of me at home. Whenever there were guests I would hide. I preferred to be in the kitchen helping Mum, rather than being with visitors. Even with my brothers, I hardly ever spoke. And with my father, the only communication I ever had was my Quran lessons, or the odd barked order.

From the very first I loved school and tried to do well in class. This was largely because school was a much happier place than home. The headmaster was called Bill Hicks. He had wild, curly brown hair and a big moustache. His brown eyes were sparkly and smiling. He taught PE, and he was a trained football referee. In his spare time he refereed for several local football clubs.

Each morning Mr Hicks would sit on a chair at the front of the school assembly hall and tell us a story, his strong, booming voice needing no microphone. Mr Hicks's tales were about everything and anything: growing up in a nearby town; going fishing in the rivers as a lad; playing football with his childhood friends; hiking with his dad in the hills; or going on an expedition to the seaside.

We were all of us captivated, even though a lot of the children were from a background similar to my own. We couldn't relate directly to what Mr Hicks was saying, for we'd never had experiences like the ones he described. His childhood, and especially his relationship with his parents, was alien to us. It was as if he was telling us about a different world to the one that we inhabited, but that just made it all the more magical and thrilling.

There was no particular lesson at the end of Mr Hicks's stories. They were a window onto another world, and perhaps that was as much as he hoped we would take away with us. But I could hardly go home and say to my parents: 'Why don't we go fishing, hiking or walking, like Mr Hicks did when he was a kid? Or on visits to the seaside? Why can't we do those things?'

I would never have dreamt of asking, for I feared the response from my father. In any case, no one did such things in our community. I knew I would be ridiculed or worse if I asked. I decided that the life of carefree fun that Mr Hicks described was what white people did, and not for us.

Neither of my parents ever told us stories about their own childhoods, and nor did they play with us. Mum used to read us the story of the Hare and the Tortoise, which she had in Urdu. But she did this to help us learn Urdu, rather than to entertain us.

The nearest we got to made-up stories was when Mum told us tales about 'bad' little girls. Invariably, they had run off on their own, told lies, argued with their siblings, or disobeyed their elders. The girls were always caught and punished by nameless, faceless monsters. And they deserved it too, Mum said.

These were morality tales, told to frighten us into being good little girls – just like my parents and the community wanted. Mum used to tell us those stories in bed. They were very different from Mr Hicks's tales of fun and adventure. But I didn't need such scary stories made up for me. Thanks to Dad, I would soon be living them for real.

There is no formal system in Islam to enable someone to become a holy man or spiritual leader. My father was not the most educated man in the community, but he did have an encyclopaedic knowledge of the Quran, from learning it by rote as a boy. That was what 'qualified' him to be our Imam.

Every Monday to Friday at 4.30 pm a white minibus would rattle down our street. 'Time to go to the mosque!' the driver would shout in Punjabi. I dreaded hearing that call. The mosque was cold, dark, damp and frightening, and our Quran teacher was cruel. I feared it and I hated it, and all my instincts told me to hide.

The mosque was actually a converted municipal library. It was strictly segregated between the sexes, having different rooms for male and female worshippers.

An arched doorway led into the men's prayer hall – a comfortable room with a wall-to-wall floral carpet. Another arched doorway led to the women's room, which was not so comfortable. Instead of a carpet, it had a few threadbare rugs scattered on the floor. If I was lucky, I would get to sit on one of those. If not, I would sit on the concrete floor.

The mosque was always freezing. The radiators were rarely switched on. Our Quran teacher would have a portable electric fire to keep her warm, but its feeble warmth wasn't enough to reach us. By the end of the hour-long lesson, our body heat plus the single electric bar might have lifted the temperature just above freezing.

Our community had purchased this building from the council. It was owned by the community, and administered by a committee of some two-dozen men, most of whom were fairly wealthy. It is seen as being 'honourable' to donate money to a mosque. Donors would have their names mentioned approvingly by the committee, and the committee's wives would ensure that news of the donation quickly circulated. This in turn allowed the donor to walk tall in the community.

Donations had been used to fund the addition of an ablution block, where worshippers could wash before prayers. There has to be running water for Muslims to perform ritual *wudu* – cleansing – before prayers. First you had to wash your face and clean your nostrils, then behind and inside your ears, followed by your neck and your arms – making sure you washed the right before the left. After that you washed your feet, in between your toes and your ankles. And finally, you washed your hands.

As you washed you would be saying the *bismillah* – the central prayer of Islam: 'There is no God but God, and Mohammed is his messenger.' We were also supposed to say the *bismillah* before entering or leaving a room, or before we ate. My father would teach the boys, while we girls went to the women's room. Our teacher was a fierce old woman, and we never got to know her name. We wouldn't dare ask what it was. We just put up our hands and waited till she looked at us. Between ourselves, we just called her 'The Teacher'.

We removed our shoes and knelt on the hard floor with a flat bench in front of us. That's how we spent the entire hour of our

Quran lessons at the mosque. The bench was for the Quran to sit on, and a book containing the Arabic alphabet. If anyone forgot either, she would get beaten with a cane. Like my father, Teacher was strict. Where he kept a broom handle by his side, she had her bamboo cane.

One time I really needed the toilet. I couldn't wait. I put my hand up.

'Yes?' Teacher snapped. 'What is it, girl?'

'May I go to the toilet, please?'

Teacher was furious at my 'lack of self-control'. 'Come here, girl! You should have gone at home!'

She took up her cane and whacked me across the palm, leaving a stinging red mark. I had been thoroughly humiliated in front of my friends, and I burst into tears. Finally, she did then let me go to the loo. But after that the others were so scared that they actually wet themselves rather than ask to be excused. That made things even worse. Teacher would always find out, and then they'd get beaten for having peed themselves.

Each of us had to learn a verse of the Quran in Arabic, repeating it over and over until we had it perfect. As the Imam's daughter, I wasn't allowed to miss a single session. But I hated the mosque lessons, and our Teacher, and I didn't ever want to go.

One day when I heard the call from the van I crawled under my bed to hide. I stayed there, barely daring to breathe, my heart beating fast. I was terrified at my own rebellion. Eventually, Dad stormed into the bedroom, grabbed me and dragged me out.

'What are you doing?' he yelled at me. '*Masjid ki gari aiya* – it's time to go to the mosque! Get in the van!'

I didn't dare argue. Another time I tried hiding in my brother Zakir's room. I didn't think Dad would find me there. But of course he did, and he was even more enraged. Then I took to hiding in the wardrobe. I'd hear various doors slamming, before he flung open the wardrobe door and went to grab me. I'd try to avoid him by swerving past, running down the stairs and bolting for the van.

Not all parents made their children go to the mosque lessons.

Amina and Ruhama got out of it by pretending they had head-aches. Their parents weren't particularly strict, and they didn't seem to mind. I was so envious of them. But my father rode up front in the minibus, and he would keep a close watch on who went and who didn't. If Amina and Ruhama missed more than one mosque session, he would go and have words with their parents.

Because my father was the Imam, he felt that he was at one with the mosque. I knew that by hiding, I was not just defying the mosque – I was also defying *him*. And for my father, such defiance was insufferable.

Such defiance would have to be punished.

Chapter Four

A Child Alone

Mum could speak only a tiny bit of English, but still far more than Dad. She could say:

'Hello, how are you?'

'How are your children?'

'How is your mother?'

Mum's only opportunity to speak English was when she picked me up from school. She could understand some of what the other mothers said, and with a shrug and a nod she could get by. With Jane and Susan's mother she tried hard to make up for her lack of words with smiles.

On one level there was precious little need for Mum to speak English. The only time she was away from the street was at school, and the weekly supermarket shop, at Morrisons. Even there she could simply fill the trolley with what she wanted, and proceed to the checkout. But Mum *wanted* to speak more. She *wanted* to be able to chat more with the school mums. She *wanted* to be able to talk to the Armenian woman across the road. She had a desire to learn, which my father did not.

Whenever we watched EastEnders and Coronation Street, Mum would try repeating what the actors said. She could tell that the characters had different accents, and she'd imitate them: doing a Cockney for EastEnders, and a Mancunian in Corrie. Her speciality was doing Ricky and Bianca, from EastEnders. Ricky was a car mechanic. He worked for one of the Mitchell brothers, the likeable villains played by Steve McFadden and Ross Kemp. He was forever shouting for his wife:

'Bianca! Bianca!'

Mum tried to copy the way he cried 'Bianca' with a nasal sound in place of the 'c'. It was hilarious when Mum yelled out, 'Bianca! Bianca!' – hearing the mixture of rural Punjabi meets East End accent that came out of her mouth. Mum didn't mind us laughing. In fact, she liked making us laugh. Deep down there was a bit of a joker in Mum.

One day Mr Hicks, the school headmaster, announced that a teacher was offering to do home lessons for families struggling to learn English. The teacher's name was Edith Smith, and she helped the kids with low reading ages at school. I introduced Mum to her, and on the spur of the moment Mum agreed that Edith could come around to teach her English.

As far as I knew, Edith Smith was the first white Englishwoman ever to enter the Shah family home. Mum had asked her round at a time when she knew Dad would be at the mosque. He spent his every afternoon there, plus all of Friday, which is the Muslim holy day. Edith was thin as a rake, and so tall than she towered over us. As a family we are fairly short in stature. She had curly brown hair, wire-rimmed glasses, and was dressed in a floral skirt and blouse. She looked like the typical English schoolmistress, but she wasn't strict or authoritarian. In fact, having Miss Smith visit was really quite fun.

That first time she smiled and ruffled my hair. 'Hello, Hannan. How are you?'

I gazed up at her and smiled back, shyly. 'Hello,' I said.

Miss Smith had brought a bag of pear drops with her, and she handed them around. They were delicious. That first English lesson was held in the back lounge. I wanted to watch in part because I was curious and in part because I just knew it was going to be fun. In no time Mum was grinning happily, as she tried to pronounce the English words.

After a while Mum offered Edith some tea. Mum's idea of 'tea' consisted of curry and chapattis, followed by biscuits and a fruit salad of apples, pears and watermelon. For a while Edith picked at the curry, trying to be polite. But she was gradually turning a brighter and brighter shade of red. Suddenly, she grabbed a glass of water and gulped it down in one go. I guess she'd bitten into a chilli!

Mum didn't seem to notice Miss Smith's discomfort, for the next time she came Mum served her yet more curry. I began bringing out a whole jug of water for poor Miss Smith. I started counting how many mouthfuls it would be before she went for that first glass of water!

Eventually, Mum must have realised that Miss Smith wasn't a fan of curry. Mum found it so funny that she'd been eating it just to be polite, while steam shot out of her ears. She told all of her friends on the street, and they found it hilarious. I must admit that I did too. Fancy not liking my mum's curry! What did white people eat at home, if not curry? Probably burgers, chips and pizza, like everyone seemed to do in EastEnders.

Of course, Mum didn't tell Dad that she had Miss Smith coming round to teach her English. And she could trust the other women on the street to stay silent about such things. Like Mum, they all had aspects of their lives that they had to keep hidden from their men, and they had an unspoken pact never to tell. It was as near as my mother ever came to a 'sisterhood'.

With each visit Mum and Miss Smith were getting to know each other better and better. They seemed able to understand each other, even though they often didn't have the right words. When the words weren't there, they used sign language and gestures. They would laugh a lot, and tease each other as if they were old friends.

When the time came for Miss Smith's lesson, Mum would bustle about happily, tidying the lounge and fetching the exercise book in which she wrote her lessons. She had to keep that book hidden amongst her sewing things. She was scared Dad would find it, and discover what she was doing. Mum's sewing machine had a cloth cover, and she kept the book tucked beneath that. Dad only ever came into the kitchen to wash before prayers, and he never looked around. To him, the kitchen was a place for women.

Normally, Mum looked tired and careworn. She wasn't exactly

full of the joys of life, which was hardly surprising when you considered what her life consisted of. Miss Smith brought a ray of light into our home, and into Mum's world. She taught Mum the alphabet, so she could write her name in English. She had to teach her to write from scratch. After that, she started with a book that went: 'A is for Apple'; 'B for Ball'; 'C for Cat', and so on.

Then they moved on to conversational English, which basically meant chatting.

'How are you?' Miss Smith asked.

'I am fine, thank you,' Mum replied.

At first she was stilted and mumbling. I could tell that she was lacking in confidence and embarrassed. But with Edith's encouragement, they were soon striking up fine conversations.

'How did you sleep?'

'I slept very well.'

'How many children do you have?'

'I have six children.'

'Are you married?'

My mum smiled, embarrassedly. What a thing to ask! Of course she was married. How could she have six children and not be?

'Yes, I am married.'

'Where do your children go to school?'

And so it went on. Eventually, it was Mum's turn to question Miss Smith.

'Are you married?' she asked.

'Yes, I have a husband,' Edith answered.

But then she explained that actually, she didn't have a husband at all. They both burst out laughing. Edith was around forty years old, and in our culture being unmarried at that age was inconceivable. The first question you always asked a Pakistani woman was: 'Are you married?' If she answered no, the next question was: 'Why aren't you married?'

But Mum never asked Miss Smith that question. She would have been quite happy to ask that of someone from her own background, but she would have needed to know Miss Smith a lot better before she could broach such a personal question. And sadly, she would never get the opportunity to know Miss Smith that well.

After Miss Smith had left I would help Mum practise the English alphabet and numbers, and try to engage her in basic conversation. After those visits, Mum would be noticeably happier. She was actually very clever, if only she'd been given a chance. Mum was like a caged bird. All she wanted was a chance to fly.

It was all going very well until one day when Dad came home early from the mosque. As usual, Mum and Miss Smith were in the lounge with me. My brothers were around, but Mum had asked them not to mention Edith's visits to Dad.

We heard the front door open and shut. It was odd, because it was the wrong time of day for anyone to be visiting. Mum immediately tensed up. A moment later the door opened and in walked Dad. He sat down on the sofa, and for a moment he almost failed to notice Miss Smith. But then he glanced up and caught sight of this white English woman in his home. Instantly, his face darkened like a thundercloud. He said not a word to Miss Smith, nor made a gesture to acknowledge her presence.

'Hello,' said Miss Smith, trying to smile a welcome at him.

He just scowled back at her and buried his head in his Quran. Miss Smith did her best to carry on with the lesson, but a dark and menacing atmosphere had seeped into the room. Mum looking terrified. She wasn't laughing and joking with Miss Smith any more.

When the lesson ended, Mum saw Edith out and went straight into the kitchen. But Dad jumped up and followed her in there. Immediately I heard shouting.

'*What are you doing?* Bringing that *gori* into the house? A dirty *gori* infidel! *In my house!* How dare you!'

Gori is the female version of gora. From where I was sitting in the lounge I heard that first, sickening thump as he hit her. Mum cried out in pain, and started crying. But Dad had no mercy. He beat her again and again.

I didn't know where he was beating her, but it was very likely to be around the body. The face would mark, and then people would know for sure what Dad was up to. In our community it wasn't acceptable for a husband to savagely assault his wife. The odd slap was fine, to keep the women in line. But beating them up just wasn't 'honourable'. If Dad were found out it would bring shame on the family. I'm sure Dad knew this, and that's why he always beat Mum where he knew it wouldn't show.

My brothers were upstairs. They must have been able to hear Mum's screams, but they didn't react. They backed Mum up whenever they could, but not when it came to Dad's violence. I guess they didn't feel they could challenge my father's authority in the family, or within the wider community as a whole.

I sat in the lounge, feeling sick with worry for my mum. Only minutes earlier she had been laughing happily with Miss Smith over her awful pronunciation. Now, for that simple, innocent pleasure she was being savagely beaten by my dad. I didn't try to intervene. I was only five years old and I was too scared to do so. Finally, Dad stormed into the men's lounge, shutting himself in there in a silent rage.

I crept into the kitchen to see what state Mum was in. She had collapsed onto the floor and she was sobbing hysterically. She didn't seem able to get up. She stayed there for several minutes, shaking with shock and pain. I tried to put my tiny arms around her, but she pushed me away. She was ashamed and embarrassed that she had been beaten, and for her little daughter to see her like this again.

I stood there bewildered, not knowing what to do. I wanted so much to help Mum, to comfort her and make her life happy – as it had been a few minutes ago. But the only way I could see of doing so was to stop Dad from hitting her. I knew it was only a matter of time before he found another excuse to beat Mum. Yet how could I, a five-year-old girl, stand in the way of my father?

I remember thinking that Dad was evil. How could he do this to Mum – my gentle, funny mother who never hurt anyone? Dad had really, really beaten her this time, and I was sure he knew exactly what he was doing. He knew where to hit Mum to ensure that the damage wasn't visible. It was planned. It was deliberate. Dad was evil.

After a few minutes more Mum slowly got to her feet, supporting herself on the work surfaces as she did so. Once again, she tried to ignore what had happened and carry on as if everything was normal. And once again, no one in the house said a word.

A few weeks later Mum and I were serving Dad his dinner in the lounge. But today was going to prove to be one of his bad days. He took one mouthful of the food, yelled out in rage, and threw the plate against the wall. It landed with a deafening crash, and then Dad started yelling at us about how disgusting it was.

'But what's wrong?' Mum asked, timidly. 'I've reheated the curry from yesterday. You liked it then . . .'

'It's cold!' Dad snarled. 'You think I want cold curry? How many years . . .'

An instant later Dad was on his feet and hitting Mum, right in the middle of the lounge. Without thinking, I went and forced my way between them.

'You're not hitting Mummy!' I cried out. I held up my arms to try to stop him. 'Stop it! Stop it! Leave Mummy alone!'

For a second Dad just stood there in utter surprise, and then he turned his angry, hate-filled eyes on me. He thumped me in the stomach. I doubled over in pain, but I stayed in front of Mum trying to protect her.

Mum was cowering behind me, seemingly frozen in shock by my resistance. Dad tried to shove me out of the way, but from somewhere I seemed to find superhuman strength and clung onto Mum. Dad started laying into me then, punching me all over the body.

'Get out of the way!' he screamed. 'I do what I like in this house! I'm your father! You do as I say! Get out of the way!'

I had started to cry, but I kept repeating the same words through my tears: 'You're not hitting Mummy. You're not hitting Mummy. You're not hitting . . .'

Finally, Dad grabbed me and threw me across the room. I was only a little girl and I wasn't very heavy. Luckily, the couch broke my fall. Without another word he stormed off into the men's room in a towering rage. As for Mum, she ran off into the kitchen to hide. Someone in the family had finally stood up to the bully, my father. Someone had finally stood up for Mum, and she was terrified what the consequences might be.

I was left alone on the couch, in tears. I stayed there for quite a while. I was so scared of what I'd done. I hadn't thought about it much. It had been a wholly instinctive reaction to stand in front of my father and take the blows intended for Mum. I was in a lot of physical pain, and I didn't feel able to move. Eventually, I must have fallen asleep, or perhaps I passed out, overwhelmed with the shock and trauma of it all.

I came to a little later. It was the sound of my brothers watching television that had brought me back to the land of the living. No one paid the slightest attention to me, or asked if I was all right. The household had reverted to its 'as-if-nothing-has-happened' mode. No one ever said anything about that first time that Dad beat me, and I never once mentioned it to Mum.

What I had done was break the unwritten rules of the household – that no one ever acknowledged Dad's violence against Mum, let alone challenged it. But I was only five years old, and I didn't know if I would dare break the rules again. In the cold light of day, perhaps the normal way of doing things was the only way to survive. But the normal way of doing things was letting Dad beat up Mum, and that I couldn't bear to live with.

In fact, the normal way of doing things had already changed. It was never going to go back to being 'normal'. My instinctive act of resistance had changed it all, for ever. From now on, instead of hitting Mum when the food wasn't 'right', Dad decided to hit me. If the house wasn't perfectly clean, I'd get a beating. I became the object of his aggression.

To start with, he beat me about once a month. But gradually, it became more often. Worse still, Mum didn't try to intervene. She was just relieved that he wasn't hitting her. Each time he beat me she acted as if nothing had happened. And it was my mother's lack of care or concern for me that really broke my heart.

Whenever he hit me, Dad would abuse me verbally: 'You're stupid, lazy and useless! You're an ugly, worthless daughter!'

There was no point in my answering back, because everyone would pretend not to hear my cries, and no one would come to help. After that first beating, I never screamed again. I just went silent whenever the blows started raining down on me.

It was a lonely time. No one was defending me. The only way that I could deal with the beatings was to go into a different world – a land of make-believe. I would imagine that I was calling out for the Loneliness Birds to come and rescue me – my magical, imaginary saviours. To either side of me their soft white wings would lift me up, and with the barest of flaps we would rise into the air, my hands gripping tightly to their downy feathers.

The Loneliness Birds were giant white doves, and they would fly down from the heavens to rescue me. Perched beside me with their wise grey eyes, they would coo soft reassurances in my ear. 'Oooh coulah . . .' This was their language, but I had been given the gift of understanding. 'Climb up . . . Climb up . . .' they were urging me. *Let us fly you away.* They would bend their legs and let me clamber onto their backs.

The Loneliness Birds would take me to a beautiful field bathed in sunshine. It was a sea of purple flowers, and as we sank towards it the wonderful smell of lavender rose to greet me. The Loneliness Birds would set me down in the Lavender Fields, where it was quiet and peaceful and secure. Here I could run around, laugh and play, and be happy and free. The white doves would stay and watch over me – like the doting, loving parents that I never had. I played alone in those fields. I was happy to play alone. In the Lavender Fields there were no other humans to abuse or hurt me.

Whenever Dad beat me I would transport myself to this other world. This was how I insulated myself from it all. Once Dad had stopped thumping me, my body would shut down and I would fall asleep, lost in my dreams of a lonely paradise. Of course, paradise couldn't last for ever. Sometime later, I would come to in the real world. Then, my tear-stained face and aching body would remind me of what had happened, and the pain and horror of it all would come flooding back to me.

As time went by my dad's beating became the norm. Whenever he struck me I started thinking to myself: *Here we go again. How long will it be to the next time?* There were bruises all over my body, but these were ignored by everyone in my family. And they were always covered by my shalwar kamiz in front of my brothers.

Once or twice, when I was getting changed for PE at school, Jane noticed and asked me about all the bruising. I told her I had fallen down the stairs. I was embarrassed and ashamed. I didn't want my best friend to treat me like a freak and ostracise me. I was lonely enough as it was. I couldn't afford to risk losing Jane.

At home nobody talked about it. Mum allowed it to happen, because if I took the abuse then she didn't get beaten herself. In our culture, it would have been difficult for Mum to do anything anyway. It would have affected the whole community. Dad was their Imam – their revered holy man. Would they have believed her if she said that he was beating his five-year-old daughter? Even if they did, would they then conclude that she'd brought shame on the family, if not the entire community, by speaking out?

In our culture, Mum could easily get the blame, and the shame, for standing up to Dad over his beating me. It is invariably considered better for a woman to suffer in silence, than to bring shame on the community. Shame had to be avoided at all costs. Anything – even child abuse – is preferable to shame. And for my mum, the family's honour was likely more important than the happiness and wellbeing of her daughter.

At first, Dad was beating me because in his warped mind there were things that I wasn't doing right: usually his food, or the cleaning. But it wasn't long before he started beating me on a whim. He struck out at me for no reason and totally unpredictably. But worse was yet to come. It would not be long before merely punishing me with a beating was not enough to satisfy Dad.

There were worse evils that he had in mind for his five-year-old daughter.

Chapter Five

Innocence Lost

Jane and Susan were the first friends I had that were not like the people on my street. Children see people's skin colour, but they don't judge them for it. At junior school we treated each other the same, no matter the hue of our skin or the colour of our hair.

To me, my two white friends had the most amazing life. They would tell me about their holidays to the seaside, their trips abroad, and their visits to relatives in different parts of the country. They never seemed to get beaten by their parents, or had to worry about bringing shame on the community. And they certainly didn't seem to spend their time double-guessing what the 'rules' might be. Jane and Susan weren't living in darkness and fear. I wanted to have their lives.

Their mum was forever inviting me to their house, to play. The invitation would come as we walked home from school. But Mum would always say that I wasn't allowed to go. She'd speak to me in Punjabi, telling me what I should say to their mum.

'Tell them you're sorry but you can't go. Tell them it's because you have to cross a very dangerous road to get there.'

'But I can go,' I'd argue with her. 'I *can* cross that road. Please let me go.'

'No. It isn't possible. Now, just tell them what I told you.'

And so I'd make my sorry excuses, and Jane's mother would smile and say maybe next time. Of course, I knew Mum's real reason for not letting me go. If Dad knew I had been to visit my white friends, he'd get mad. Dad chose to believe that white people were dirty, godless and immoral. They might even give

49

you pork to eat. If any one of us set foot in a gora's house, we could be contaminated or corrupted.

I didn't argue with Mum. I knew Dad was the reason. But once every week I would keep telling her that I wanted to go to visit them. Mum's response was always the same – *it wasn't allowed*. Of course, Jane and Susan kept inviting me. They could see no reason why they couldn't have their cute brown friend over to play.

'Come on,' Jane would say. 'Come and play at our house! We've got Barbies and everything. And we can all get into our swimming stuff and go in the pool.'

Well, I knew that I absolutely wasn't allowed to go swimming. Swimming meant showing forbidden flesh – bare ankles, arms and thighs. Dad wouldn't allow that, even though I was just a small child. Swimming lessons had started at school, but my parents had written a note saying that I couldn't go. At first they used the reason that I didn't have a swimsuit. They also said I had problems with my hearing, and couldn't get my ears wet.

In fact they dictated the letter to me in Urdu, and got me to write it out in English. My dad was too smart to say outright that I couldn't go swimming because I wasn't allowed to show any flesh. He knew that the teachers wouldn't understand, or accept, that little girls weren't allowed to show bare skin.

But still the teachers tried to find a way around his excuses. They didn't want me to be the odd one out. From somewhere they found me a swimsuit, and a hat to protect my ears. But my parents just reacted by insisting that I wasn't allowed to go swimming. They had run out of convincing reasons, so they just said point blank that I wasn't allowed. And the teachers felt that they couldn't go against them.

I never did get to go. Instead, when everyone else went to the pool, I was left in the classroom doing some colouring. Some-times there would be other kids with me. Maybe one or two would be ill with a cold or flu. But they at least had a reason. I was the freak who just wasn't allowed.

Of course, if I had gone swimming all my bruising would have shown. That I am sure was another, unspoken reason for my parents to forbid it. But as with everything in our lives, it was disguised under the cloak of 'Islam' as being *haram* – forbidden. And with my father being the Imam, who was going to challenge his version of what was allowed?

Mum said that the real reason for the swimming ban was so that no one would see my body. She chose to live by the lies of my father. Things were easier that way. I always had to keep my legs and arms covered anyway – that was what shalwar kamiz did for us. When everyone else wore a skirt or shorts for PE lessons, I had to wear shalwar kamiz trousers. Once again, I was the school weirdo.

There were other Pakistani Muslims at the school, so there were other kids who wore shalwar kamiz. But the other Muslim parents allowed their kids to go swimming. Some of the girls wore cotton trousers in the pool, to cover their legs. So like a lot of the rules my father set, the ban on swimming didn't make any sense – unless it was to hide the evidence of the beatings he was subjecting me to.

Whenever Dad beat me he would rant on and on about how 'unwanted' I was. He'd never wanted a daughter, he said, and I would never be good enough for his God, *Allah*. The gates of heaven would never open for a worthless girl like me. I was going straight to hell, and my father was about to take me there.

Some six months after that first beating, the style of the abuse changed horribly. That day, Dad had already beaten me, and called me all the usual names. I had retreated to my bedroom, and lost myself in sunny visions of the Lavender Fields.

All of a sudden the door creaked open and my father stepped into the room. This was unheard of in our house. Dad never entered into the women's bedroom. This was where Mum and I slept, and he never came in here. I shrank under the blanket in a desperate attempt to hide and avoid another beating. He stared at me, an expression of loathing mixed with something else on his bearded face.

'You – you're evil,' he announced, quietly. 'You will surely burn in hell. But for now, your evil must be punished, driven out of you. Beating isn't enough . . .'

He stepped towards me, murmuring over and over that I was a 'dirty, worthless, temptress girl' and that he'd 'never wanted a daughter'. He stopped by the bed. I had my eyes clamped shut, willing the Loneliness Birds to carry me away. I felt his hand reaching for the blanket. My body tensed up as he tugged it away from me. All of a sudden he was fumbling, roughly, with my clothes.

When I was naked he forced his hands between my legs, and started touching me. I was terrified. He was breathing heavily and his eyes were on fire. I can still remember his horrid smell. What was happening? What was he doing? He kept on telling me that he was punishing me. His breath was harsh as he kept on touching me, again and again. It hurt, but not as much as the beatings. But somehow it felt worse: I knew it was wrong and nasty and dirty.

The he lifted up his own shalwar kamiz. I felt him grab my hand and drag it roughly towards him. He forced my fingers around his flesh.

'This is the way to punish an evil, worthless girl like you,' he gasped. 'Just look at you, doing it . . . Look how dirty you are.'

He started moving my hand upon him. I kept my eyes clamped shut in fear and disgust, but still I could smell him. I knew it was his thing I was holding, and I felt physically sick, consumed by loathing – for myself as much as for him. All of the time he kept gasping about how evil and ugly I was, and how I was getting the punishment a dirty girl like me deserved.

I did what my dad demanded of me. I took my punishment. How could I do otherwise? I was a confused and terrified little girl, and part of me still wanted his approval and his love. In my mind, I hated him for doing this to me. But in my heart there was still a part of me that wanted him to love me as a father should. I acquiesced in his demands, hoping that it would somehow make him love me. But Dad was not interested in love. This just made him loathe me all the more. I was 'tempting' him by not resisting, and so I was the guilty evil temptress his mind wanted me to be.

He hitched up his robes. 'You deserve everything you got,' he sneered. 'And if you ever tell anyone about your punishment, I will kill you. And then you'll go to hell. Allah would never allow a dirty girl like you into Paradise.'

My father was only interested in power and control, and in satisfying his own sick desires. He had realised that he had total power over me, and he had become intoxicated by it. He could do whatever he wanted. He knew no one was going to defend me or stop him.

He left me on the bed, terrified, and wracked with guilt and shame. I believed what he had told me. If someone tells you something often enough, you start to believe it, especially when that person is your father. And it is even more the case when your father just happens to be the universally respected Imam.

It seemed that Dad rapidly developed a taste for this abuse. The next week, the same thing happened. And the next week. And the week after that. It was as if my father couldn't keep his hands off me. I never knew exactly when it would happen next, and I dreaded it. I lived in a state of constant fear.

But Dad wasn't content for long only with touching. The first time that he raped me, I felt as if I was going to die from the agony of his weight pushing down on me. He left me bleeding all over the bed. I had to lie to Mum and tell her that I'd had a nosebleed. How a nosebleed ended up bloodying the bed halfway down the sheets didn't seem to matter to Mum. She just scolded me for dirtying the bed and making more work for her to do.

Soon, the rapes had become routine. He would take me into the bedroom for 'punishment', and I'd stare at the ceiling pretending it was happening to someone else. And I'd hope and pray for the Loneliness Birds to carry me away to my world of make-believe, where my rapist father couldn't touch me any more.

'You are evil,' was my dad's catchphrase. 'And this is the only way to drive the evil out of you.'

Each time he raped me, I felt more and more disgusting and dirty. I was spending more and more time away in my world of make-believe, but not even that could shield me from the horror and shame of it all. I felt dirty and worthless and sick to the core of my soul. I believed that I deserved my 'punishment'. But when would it ever end?

Incredibly, Mum never once questioned my nosebleed stories. For the first few weeks I bled every time, so it must have been obvious what was going on. I could hardly be having a nosebleed every week, and always halfway down the bed. Mum seemed unable to defend me when he beat me, and unable to defend me now. She didn't want to face the truth. It would have been too shameful for her. She would rather have died. It would have destroyed our 'honour', and our family.

There was no one I could talk to about it, no one I could confess to. My family didn't want to know. I wasn't close to my teachers. Other than my friends, I was completely alone. Mostly, I felt enough of a misfit already at school. I wasn't about to reveal to my friends this new and unspeakable horror. And, at five years old pushing six, I didn't have the words to explain to anyone, even had I wanted to.

Instead, I started to make up stories in my head. I imagined for myself a different life, hoping I could make it real. I started inventing stories about being a little white girl, living in Jane and Susan's house, or even being their sister. In my tortured child's mind, being white, and having what I thought was a normal life and a normal, loving family, were inextricably linked. It was young Muslim girls of Pakistani origin like me whose lives were hell.

I started to write some of the stories down in a little notebook I kept hidden on top of the wardrobe. I wrote in English, so that even if my parents found them they wouldn't know what they were about. In that sense, English was my secret, code language, but it was also the language of the family and the community that I dreamed about joining. I escaped into the life of white people, for I could never imagine any of my father's horrors happening in Jane and Susan's world.

I could do nothing to stop my father, and did as he demanded – no matter how sick and revolting it made me feel. It was a vicious circle. The more the abuse went on, the more dirty and deserving of such punishment I felt. The more my father got away with it, the more dark and abusive his power trip became. Within many Islamic societies, a victim of rape is often seen as the guilty party, having somehow tempted the man into sexual excess. And likewise, my father blamed me for 'tempting' him into the abuse.

Eventually he was no longer sated by the hurried rapes in the bedroom. Or perhaps it was because the bloodied sheets were becoming hard to explain away. Either way, he decided to take me to a new place of torture. At the back of the house, beneath the kitchen, lay a cellar. And this was to become the place of my abuse for the next ten years.

Through a wooden door and down some creaky wooden steps was a dark and damp brick cell, about the size of a small and narrow bedroom. Bare brick walls. A bare brick floor. No light bulb, just a stained and half-rotten standard lamp casting a dim, eerie glow. The cellar wasn't used for anything much, and there were vermin that would scamper across the floor. Dad could lock the door and do whatever he wanted to me in there, at his leisure and without the slightest danger of being disturbed.

My father took to locking me down there, with no food and no water. He kept me imprisoned there for hours on end – sometimes even for days – naked in the cold and damp. I had nothing to keep me warm other than just the shalwar kamiz I had been wearing when he dragged me down there to be 'punished'.

'You! Don't you know no man will ever want you!' he kept taunting me. 'You're disgusting and dirty. Look at you! You'll never be married because you are a useless, dirty, worthless girl.'

Once he was done with raping me he would leave me down there, alone and shivering in the suffocating dark. Mice and unseen things scuttled around me, as I huddled against one brick wall. This was my living nightmare. I hunched myself into a corner wishing I was dead, and praying for the Loneliness Birds to come rescue me. I dreamed of them carrying me off into a land populated by noble princes and beautiful princesses.

In my mind I was one of them – and all in this world were white. They lived in castles surrounded by fields of lavender, and they had everything one could wish for. Everything was happy and everything was good. But this magical world couldn't hold me for ever, and eventually I would come to my senses. Those times were the worst of all. It was then that I would wish for my life to end, and for an end to the darkness and suffering.

Sometimes, Dad would go to the mosque to spend the afternoon sermonising to his flock, leaving me locked in the cellar. If he'd left the key in the outside of the door, Mum might bring me some food: a plate of curry with some chapattis. But she stayed completely silent while she delivered it to the door above, wordlessly handing the plate to me. Sometimes I was only half-dressed when I came up those creaking steps, but she wouldn't even mention it, or offer me a blanket.

She wouldn't even look at me. She didn't want to acknowledge what was plain to see – that her husband, the Imam, was abusing her six-year-old daughter.

Not once did I ask her to let me out. I knew that she was too scared of Dad to release me. Once he had caught her bringing me food, and he flew into a terrible rage, beating Mum savagely. As his fists pounded her, he screamed at Mum for interrupting his 'punishment'. How could he cure my evil ways if his wife kept interfering, he ranted. He was the master of this house, and he knew what was good for his cursed daughter.

Mum was terrified of him. But a couple of times she did take the risk of leaving the door unlocked so I could escape. She just hoped that Dad thought it was his own forgetfulness not locking me in there properly. But mostly, he would return from the mosque, come down into the cellar and rape me again.

Sometimes I was left in there for days on end. I'd even miss school, but I'd just tell the teachers that I had been kept at home because I was ill. I must have looked pale and sick and exhausted. None of my teachers ever questioned it, or seemed suspicious about what was really happening at home.

*

Jane and Susan persisted in inviting me over to their house. They got their mother to up her campaign of persuasion with my mum.

'Hannan must come round to visit,' their mother remarked to mine, one day after school. 'The girls are dying to have her over. We'd love to have her. Don't you think she might?'

Mum smiled and said 'thank you', but she left it there. She avoided setting a date, or even giving a definite answer. It was always such a good excuse, hiding behind her lack of English. I decided there and then to take the next opportunity I got to sneak off to their house. I knew where it was, because we walked past it on the way home from school. If I wasn't gone for too long, Mum would just think that I was playing in a friend's house somewhere on our street.

One summer afternoon I slipped out of the house without a word of explanation. I was always off at Amina's, or another friend's house, so I knew I wouldn't be missed. I made my way down East Street until I reached the main road. It was scary, with cars zooming back and forth at breakneck speed. It took me several attempts before I finally plucked up courage and dashed across. Now Jane and Susan's house was right in front of me.

Jane and Susan lived in a big, modern-looking detached house. Whenever we had walked past I had marvelled at their front garden full of beautiful flowers. In a way, it reminded me of the Lavender Fields of my world of make-believe. I made my way along the path at the side of their house, and there were Jane and Susan, playing on the swings in the back garden. As soon as they caught sight of me they started squealing with delight.

'You made it! Wow! Hannan's here!'

I glanced around me. I could barely believe my eyes. Their back garden was even more magical and beautiful than the front. It was like something out of a fairy tale. There was a wide lawn fringed with a riot of bright flowers. Chairs and a table were arranged around a little pond. And a paddling pool complete with plastic ducks was on the far side, with buckets and spades scattered on the grass.

Jane and Susan rushed across and grabbed me by the hand,

leading me over to the pool. It was such a gorgeous sunny day and they were dressed in skimpy Lycra shorts and tops. I felt so awkward in my hot, all-enveloping shalwar kamiz. Their mum was in the kitchen. From the open window she called out a jolly greeting, and emerged with a plate of biscuits and glasses of squash to welcome me.

The three of us played outside for a bit, and then they invited me in to see their rooms. We went through the kitchen, and upstairs. Of course, their mum didn't mind one bit having me in their house. The first surprise I got was that Jane and Susan each had their own room. On the door of each was a big painted sign, announcing it to be 'Jane's Room' or 'Susan's Room'. Inside each was a pine bed high enough so you could sit underneath – and that was where they stored their toys. It was like Pandora's Box for me. I didn't have one single toy at home.

Their parents made sure they each had the same things. Each had a doll's house, with a set of wooden furniture. There were My Little Ponies, and Barbie dolls with a lavish wardrobe of clothes. Jane, Susan and I spent ages dressing the Barbies, combing their hair and driving them around in their cars. Then we each took turns combing our own hair: Susan's fire-red tresses, Jane's brunette locks and my jet-black mane. Jane had a dressing table with plastic jewellery, hairbrushes, and pretty flower hair clips.

In no time two hours had flown by, two hours of this illicit, forbidden pleasure. I started to think about going home. If I was away for much longer Mum was bound to start looking for me. It wouldn't take her long to discover that I wasn't on the street. Just about everyone knew everyone, so it wouldn't be hard to find out. Reluctantly, I said my goodbyes to Jane and Susan, and their mum.

'Come again, any time,' she told me. 'It was lovely. You had such a nice time playing together. Promise you'll come.'

'I promise,' I murmured. 'And thanks.'

I didn't know if I would be able to keep that promise. With dragging feet I retraced my steps, hoping that no one would see me. I slipped back unnoticed into my house, a place of darkness and foreboding after the light and joy of Jane and Susan's home.

'Where have you been?' were Mum's first words.

'Out playing on the street,' I replied, as innocently as I could.

I avoided her eye and busied myself in the kitchen. I knew she had work for me to do. Mum didn't ask me any more. We never spoke much in any case. And she was used to me wandering the street. It was leaving it – crossing the divide into the gora's territory – that was forbidden.

My visit to my friends' house had been true rebellion. It felt frightening and dangerous, and I was relieved that no one had actually caught me. But it was also exciting, and somehow liberating. That evening, I thought to myself that it was good to have done it. I had broken the rules, and it felt good. It was my first secret rebellion, and I would keep it all to myself. I vowed there would be more.

In the days that followed, I reflected on the differences between my life and that of Jane and Susan. I thought of all the toys they had, and the fact that they each had their own room, and the magical playground in the back garden. Why was my life like it was, and their life as it was, I wondered. Why?

But most of all I wondered why they had such a nice mum who took me into their home, when my white friends were banned from my house. She seemed so lovely: she laughed and chatted with her daughters, as if they were friends. Jane and Susan had conversations with their parents, rather than just receiving orders and abuse. Having seen the place they lived in, I'd be embarrassed to bring them home to my house. I had nothing – *absolutely nothing* – for them to play with.

I guessed their parents had to be really rich. We couldn't have afforded everything they had. No doubt about it, my parents were poor. But my brothers had toys. They didn't have very many, but they each had a few Star Wars troopers and that sort of thing. But I had nothing. How could I ever invite my friends to play? In a way, it was a relief that having white friends to visit was banned.

But still I wondered why I had no toys – not even one. I could only conclude that this was my place in life. I was not a beloved daughter, like Jane and Susan. I wasn't an honoured son, like my brothers. I was useless and shameful – to be used and abused at Dad's will.

I wanted Susan and Jane's life. I presumed that their good fortune and happy lives were somehow linked to their skin colour. In my mind, one came with the other. I didn't link it with religion. Only with race. Because they were white, I presumed they were Christian. But they didn't go to church or talk about God. In any case, it wasn't their religion I longed for – it was their parents, and their golden, sunlit lives.

To me, Jane and Susan lived in the Lavender Fields – the happy, safe place of my dreams.

Chapter Six

Submission

By now Mum had decided that it was time for me to start doing the domestic chores. I had to cook, spending a lot of time in the dismal kitchen. The walls were painted pale yellow. It had 1960s-style wooden laminate kitchen units, a red tiled floor, and a stainless steel sink. In one corner was a huge pipe that ran down the wall. The one source of light was a bare bulb hanging from the ceiling.

The first time I cooked Mum showed me how to cut the onion the way she wanted, sliced very finely. I tried to do as she wanted, but it was the first time I'd handled a knife, and my childish hands were too clumsy. I cut the onion into thickish slices and put them in the pan to fry them with the oil and spices. Mum looked over to check what I was doing. Without warning she flew into a temper.

'Weren't you listening?' she cried. 'Weren't you watching? The onions need to be smaller, just like I showed you! How can you be so stupid?'

I was shaken and shamed. I was used to such words from my father, but Mum had never spoken to me in such a nasty way. Unlike Dad, Mum didn't actively *dislike* me. Normally, she was a kindly, protective figure, although she couldn't protect me from my dad's abuses. But in the kitchen she was a tyrant. She had set ways of doing things, and she would get annoyed if they weren't done her way. Even the smallest mistake would earn me a scolding.

I lived in fear of getting it wrong. If one single thing was perceived as not being perfect with his food, that was Dad's excuse to fly into a raging fury. Mum lived in fear of that, and I suppose she took the stress out on me. Her life with Dad was so abusive and dark that she had learned some of his abusive ways herself.

Whenever I did anything 'wrong' in the kitchen, Mum assumed I had been daydreaming. In fact, I just wasn't a natural at cooking. She liked chapattis to be perfectly round to fit on the plates, and I could never make them round enough. I'd take a lump of dough, ball it up, and roll it out flat with a rolling pin. But whereas Mum's were all perfect circles, I never once managed to roll a perfect chapatti. Mine were all raggedy-edged and irregular.

Dad was forever ordering me to fetch him food and drink from the kitchen. But he was even less happy with my cooking than he was with Mum's. No matter what I cooked – chicken, okra, or vegetable curry – he would declare that it was awful, and that I was 'useless'. And with my chapattis that weren't perfectly round, he'd throw them back at me.

'What's this?!' he'd yell. 'Useless! Put it in the bin! I want round ones like your mother makes. Go and do it again. And you'd better get it right this time . . .'

There was always the fear in my mind that he might beat me, or worse still 'punish' me by dragging me into the cellar. And things only got worse after my little sister, Sabina, was born, and became old enough to help in the kitchen. She turned out to be a natural cook. She could make perfect curries, just like Mum, and perfectly round chapattis.

Sabina would show off, singing out: 'Look! Look at my round chapattis! Round – just like Dad loves them!' When she delivered them to my father he would eat them up with gusto.

I couldn't just shrug it off. I couldn't just tell myself – *a round chapatti or a square one – what's the difference? Who cares?* I wanted to be able to do it right. I wanted to please my father. I thought that this was all part of being a proper Muslim girl. But I just never seemed able to master it. The more Mum criticised me, the more nervous I became in the kitchen, forgetting to add salt or spices because my nerves had got the better of me.

As for my brothers, they never commented on my food. They just ate it up, their faces invariably glued to the telly. I was relieved that they didn't abuse me and throw it back in my face. That was compliment enough for me.

One afternoon when I was nearly seven years old, I was watching a children's cartoon called Button Moon. It was about a moon that these odd little characters lived on, which was really a giant shirt button. I loved that programme. I laughed at one of the jokes, when suddenly I heard Dad's voice from the doorway.

'Shut up!' he snapped. 'I don't *ever* want to hear you laughing. I don't even want to see you smile. Or else.'

I turned back to the TV in fear. I knew if I answered back it would be the cellar for me. But in that instant I made a vow to myself: *I am going to laugh and smile. I'll never stop, no matter what you do to me.* I was determined not to let my father take that from me. It was a part of me that I wouldn't let him violate or kill. Laughing gave me strength, and helped me to be brave. It was a part of my soul that he couldn't totally darken or destroy.

My father had all but beaten the laughter and the joy out of my mother. I never once saw her happy when he was around. But my schoolteachers often remarked that I was the easiest person to make laugh. I smiled so readily, almost because there was so little to lighten my life at home. Like an eager puppy desperate for love and kindness, it took very little to make me smile.

Even something as commonplace as a school outing to the church was a big deal for me. Bermford Parish Church was cold and cavernous, almost like a cathedral. But the vicar was lovely – a warm, friendly man in his thirties, who wore a black suit and white collar. He had started visiting the school, to help with the RE lessons. He really made the Bible stories come alive, his words painting such vivid, life-like pictures.

One day he had told us the story of baby Jesus. Another time it was the story of Joseph and his Technicolor dreamcoat, or of Moses and the burning bush, or of Daniel in the lion's den, or the story of Jesus healing the lepers. As he talked he drew cartoon-like pictures with coloured pencils on a flip-board, to help illustrate his words. He was a talented artist, and he really made those stories come alive. Sometimes he even brought puppets and would act out the Bible tales.

Sometimes, he got us to act them out in class. I never volunteered for anything. I just hid in the back, while others went forward to be sheep and shepherds and the like. Whilst he taught us about Christianity, we learned about Hinduism and Islam and other religions from the main RE teacher. The school prided itself on celebrating all religious festivals. They held special assemblies for the Muslim festival of Eid, the Hindu festival of Diwali, and the Jewish festival of Hanukah.

The vicar's were by far the best lessons, and I got the impression he really was inspired by his beliefs. His enthusiasm was infectious, and he made it all seem so enjoyable. Church visits weren't always such good fun though. I remember falling asleep in the pews. At some point during the service most pupils would nod off. For me the difference was that at the mosque you'd get beaten horribly for doing so, whereas nothing like that happened in church.

One day the vicar told us a story about Jesus. He finished off by explaining that Jesus is one of the prophets mentioned in the Quran alongside the prophet Mohammed. I was very surprised. Dad had never mentioned him before. I decided that I was going to tell Dad all about it. Maybe he would be pleased that I had found out about Jesus being in the Quran, and that Christianity and Islam shared prophets.

'The teacher told us Jesus is in the Quran,' I ventured, hopefully, once Dad got home. Maybe for once he would be pleased with me. 'He said . . .'

'Don't you ever mention THAT MAN'S name in this house!' my father roared. 'Never again, you hear me!'

And then I felt his knuckles against my face as he slapped me with the back of his hand. The stinging pain left me in no doubt that 'Jesus' was also against the rules.

It was only much later in life that I would realise that Jesus is a major prophet in Islam. In the Quran he is known by the Arabic name of 'Isa'. Perhaps Dad was ignorant of this fact, or perhaps he just hated the Christian version of the name. Whatever, no explanation was offered for my father's blind hatred of 'Jesus'.

But I carried on listening to the vicar's lessons, and I carried on smiling at his stories. That was one thing my father couldn't take away from me – my laughter. It made me feel like a survivor. He'd taken my innocence, my childhood love, and polluted it all. He'd taken my body, and abused and violated it. And he'd used his cruel words to try to destroy my soul. But he couldn't kill my laughter. That he couldn't kill.

One day I was in town with my brother Raz and Mum. We were going to Morrisons supermarket, and she wanted Raz and me to help with the shopping. We didn't have a car, so this was one of the weekly chores. Mum had a green-checked shopping trolley – the kind of thing old people use – for the heaviest things.

Just as we were about to enter the supermarket, a tall white man came up to us. He was wearing a white *jellabiya* – a Muslim robe – and a *topi* – a skullcap. This was the 'uniform' worn by my father, and the other men on our street. It looked very out of place being worn by this gora. He had a big beard dyed red with henna, and piercing blue eyes.

Raz greeted him with a manly hug, and it turned out that they knew each other from the mosque. This was the first time that I'd ever seen a white convert to Islam. Raz told us he was mightily pleased that this gora had converted, but I was surprised. Dad had never mentioned that there was a white convert at the mosque. I didn't even think white people were allowed in there. I thought they would be banned, as they were at home.

Anyway, why on earth would a white person want to leave their world and joins ours, I wondered. Over time I learned that there were other converts in Dad's mosque. White or black, they were welcomed by most people, as long as they were coming to Islam. In fact, many people in our community had friends who were 'outsiders'. My uncles would talk openly about their goray friends. It was chiefly my father who seemed to hate all outsiders.

Dad wouldn't actively scold people in the community for having 'foreign' friends. He just ignored it. In his mind there was a strict hierarchy. First came the Pakistani Muslims, especially the holy men such as himself, and the Arab Muslims. Then came other Asian Muslims – Indians, Bangladeshis and others. Next came the white unbelievers, and then the blacks. On the bottom of the pile and to be most reviled were the Jews.

In Saudi Arabia – the Muslim holy land – Pakistani Muslims are generally seen as being 'lesser' because they are not Arabs. My father was aware of this and he accepted it and his place in the pecking order. The Saudi Arabs were the direct descendants of the prophet Mohammed, and hence they were the most exalted. My father seemed to accept all of this. It was the way of the world.

In my father's mosque there was no joint place of worship for men and women. They were kept strictly segregated at all times. This total separation is not a tenet of my parents' Deobandi Sunni belief. There are joint areas of worship in many Deobandi mosques. This was my father's rule – and his rule and the mosque's rule were one and the same thing.

On Friday – the Muslim holy day – my father would spend his entire day at the mosque. Mum would be at home cooking a special meal – delicately spiced rice pudding and *halvah*, an Arabic sweet made of crushed sesame seeds and honey. Friday was the day for having a bath, and for scenting the house with incense. Dad insisted that his best clothes be made ready for him – laid out in the front room perfectly clean and perfectly pressed. If anything was out of place, woe betide Mum and me.

Sometimes, there would be special Friday events at a neighbouring mosque. A holy man – a *pir* – from Pakistan or from Saudi Arabia would come to give a lesson and to recite the Quran. The mosques would club together to pay for the pirs to fly over. There would be great excitement about the impending visit of the pir, but only the men would be allowed to attend the lesson and recital at the mosque.

The women had to content themselves with watching a video

of the event afterwards. The presence of women in the mosque might be embarrassing or distracting for the men, especially if they were pretty. The presence of a woman, even one fully shrouded in a burka, was thought to be unbearably enticing and off-putting. Any hint of femininity might detract from the men's ability to concentrate on the Quran recital, so lessening their spiritual experience.

Somehow, it never occurred to my father and the other men that they should curtail their lecherous, blinkered ways, rather than banning women from the mosque. Even though the Quran commands men to be modest as well as women, it never manifested itself in that way. It was never said that a woman might be distracted by the sight of a man. The men never had to be excluded from the mosque, whilst the pir gave a lesson to a wholly female congregation. There was no concept of equality in my father, the Imam's, world.

Each child in our community was assigned a pir. The pir would pray for the child to be strong in his or her faith, and to uphold the Five Pillars of Islam. Sometimes, the pir would come to visit the child's home. This was considered a very great honour. Houses would be scrubbed from top to bottom, and a great celebration would be planned. When the pir visited, everyone would want to touch his hand or his robe, almost as if they themselves were objects of veneration.

Pirs received cash donations from families to take on their children. There was no set rate, but it was 'honourable' to give as much as possible. Invariably, the pirs were far better off than the people to whom they ministered. They dressed in well-tailored clothes, and would come driving down the street in sleek Mercedes cars. Any man could declare that he'd been called by God to be a pir, but not a woman, of course.

When I was seven years old my pir came to visit me. He was of Pakistani origin, but he lived in Saudi Arabia. He came from a long line of pirs – it ran in the family. When he arrived at our house he swept regally into the women's lounge. My father, plus a gaggle of women including my mum, my sister and my aunties, came forward to greet him. The room quickly filled up with as many women as could fit in. Most were there just to be in his presence and to touch his robe.

He proceeded to sit on the floor, and we all followed suit. The main thing that I noticed was the pir's overpowering smell. He was wearing a heady, spicy oil. Strict Muslims believe that you shouldn't even use alcohol on the skin, as alcohol is haram. Instead, you have to use halal aftershave, or scented oil, which is difficult to find in Britain.

I was reeling from the pir's incredibly pungent smell. He began to recite parts of the Quran, and I had to follow him, line by line. He told me I had to recite those verses every day. Then he gave my parents two gifts. The first was a *taviz* – a small metal locket to put around my neck, containing one verse of the Quran handwritten by him. Common mortals are not allowed to write down the Quran, but as a pir he was allowed. The second gift was a verse written on a piece of paper. My parents were supposed to chop it up and put it in my drink, so that I would ingest the holy words into my body.

With that the ceremony was complete. I had met my pir, my spiritual guide, and for me my big day was done. Dad and the pir disappeared into the men's lounge for hours of tea and conversation.

Everyone had made such a big deal about this holy man coming to visit. I had been so looking forward to it. At last, my family were doing something to make me feel special. We were all wearing new clothes. For once, even I was dressed up. We had cleaned the whole of the house, and cooked a feast – the sort of food that we would never normally eat. Yet the pir had only been with me for two minutes, if that.

The pir had decided to eat in the men's lounge, and we women weren't allowed in there. That rule wasn't about to be relaxed just because it was supposed to be my special day. Instead, I spent my time ferrying plates of sumptuous food from the kitchen into the men's lounge. Each time I knocked on the door one of my brothers took the plates from me. Then the door was shut in my face.

Once the men had finished eating, I was allowed to eat with the women in the back lounge. I enjoyed the food, but couldn't shake the feeling that it was all such a scam. Meeting my pir had been a non-event. If that was the greatest treat that my parents could manage for me in the first seven years of my life, then they could keep it. Meeting my pir? Big deal, I told myself. Give me Jane and Susan's Barbie dolls, or their wooden doll's house and furniture, any day of the week.

Later, my mum gave me the pir's locket to wear, plus the Quran verse chopped into a glass of orange squash. I had to swallow the little pieces of paper along with the squash. If I had strained it out with my teeth, I'd have been in big trouble.

If there was a highlight to the mosque goings-on, it was wedding times. A wedding generally lasted for three days, and included a henna party, a register office signing, and two celebrations: the first at the groom's house, and the second at the bride's house. But the main ceremony took place at the mosque. If we knew the family well, we'd get invited to the henna party, at which the bride and her female friends would get their hands and feet painted.

Using a tube of henna – a traditional, plant-based dye – painters produced complicated designs: swirls, fans, tendrils, buds, and delicate flowers. When the henna dried and cracked off, the women would be left with an intricate pattern of earthy red that could last for weeks.

The henna parties also involved traditional Pakistani dancing – something similar to Bollywood dancing. It was very flirtatious, but of course the women would never do it in front of the men. The women only ever danced with other women! In Afghanistan there was a similar dance, and traditionally the men and women had performed it together. But with the coming of the Taliban men and women dancing together had been banned.

At the mosque men and women were separated for the wedding. The bride was allowed into the men's room, accompanied by her mother and aunt. She would look stunning in a pink shalwar kamiz – pink or red is the traditional colour of Muslim bridalwear – and she would glitter with jewellery. Gold bracelets would hang off her arms, gold necklaces would be threaded around her throat, and long gold earrings would dangle from her ears. And a beautiful gold pendant – a *tika* – would fall in the centre of her forehead.

She would sit on a stage alongside the groom, who would be dressed in a Western-style suit, with a waistcoat. Dad would read out the wedding ceremony, while we women and girls were locked away in our room, gossiping among ourselves. There was plenty of room to run around, so I'd have fun playing with my friends. But no singing or dancing was allowed.

Meanwhile, the bride was not supposed to smile or seem in any way happy. If ever a bride looked even remotely joyful, Dad would scold her. She was supposed to show sorrow at leaving her parents. Often, this wasn't difficult. All the marriages were arranged ones, and invariably the bride was nervous as to what lay ahead, if not downright terrified. In some cases, she wouldn't even have met the groom until she reached the register office. So naturally, the bride would sit there with a very long face. As for the groom, he was allowed to be happy if he felt like it.

Dad would ask both of them if they agreed to the marriage. Presuming they said 'yes' – and woe betide any daughter who dithered or erred – he would then get them to recite a particular Surah from the Quran. Following the ceremony, the men tucked into the wedding feast, the bride and groom remaining sitting on their stage. When the men had finished they went into a side room, and we women and girls were finally allowed in to eat.

During the feast, people went up to the couple and gave them gifts – clothes, things for the home, or envelopes full of money. Later, in the groom's house, the bride's parents put a garland of money around the groom's neck, which was part of the dowry they owed. The parents would have reached a private agreement before the wedding as to how much the dowry should be. There was no set amount, but it would usually include money, new clothes, and livestock for the extended family in Pakistan.

Part of the reason that girls are often so unwelcome in Pakistan is that it will cost their parents so much to marry them off. This is the curse of the dowry system. Not surprisingly, Dad took every opportunity to remind me that he never wanted a daughter. Our entire community valued boys more than girls. Boys were celebrated. Girls were an unwelcome burden. Parents would thank God when they got a baby boy, but there would be no such thanksgiving if it was a girl.

One day I happened to see a documentary on the television about the treatment of girls in Asia. It pointed out that in India and Pakistan, female children were seen as being so costly to the family that they were often killed at birth. Back in my father's village girls could be killed at birth, simply because they were girls.

I had thought that Dad was just a one-off in his hatred of womankind. But now the pieces began to fall into place for me. The whole of our culture seemed geared against women and girls. I felt very angry, but at the same time part of me felt as if I should have been one of those girls murdered at birth. It seemed all I had achieved by surviving was to become a victim of my father.

Not every father in our community was like mine. Plenty of them did show love to their children, daughters as well as sons. There were other dads in the street that played with their kids: kicking a football around, or even holding a skipping rope for the girls. I'd seen Amina and Ruhama's father, Abdul, being lovely to them. He would play chase with them in the park, and he would even sit and help them do their homework.

If Amina, Ruhama and I were playing hide and seek, their father might play with us, searching for me if it was my time to hide. He used to cuddle Amina and Ruhama, and tickle them while they giggled happily. Abdul didn't hug me or tickle me, but he was always nice to me. Whenever I went to their house, he would be kind and friendly: 'Hello, Hannan!' he'd say. 'How are you? How are your parents?'

By contrast, Dad never had a real conversation with any small

71

child. When my brothers got old enough, he would talk to them – but only about mosque business, or news from Pakistan or the Middle East. There was never any warmth, laughter or affection. Dad never hugged anyone in our house, not even his own wife.

The only physical contact from him came in the darkness of the nightmare.

Chapter Seven

My Father's House

I hear him before I see him, mumbling away to himself in Punjabi.

I am in the cellar again. I am lying on the floor, naked. There is the standard lamp that casts that dim, eerie glow. Other than that it is dark and cold as the grave. It is by the light of the lamp that I see him. I am terrified. I am gripped by fear. I can sense the stiffness and tension in my entire body.

Yet at the same time it's like it's not my body, but someone else's. He's not doing this to *me*. It's someone else lying here in the dirt and shadows.

I wait for him to decide what he wants to do with me. I am eight years old, and somehow I still live in hope. Hope that he'll release me and stop. Hope that someone will save me. But no one ever comes.

I hear shuffling feet, sandals moving across the bare brick floor. He is moving towards me. I don't want to breathe. I don't what to show him that I'm *alive* even. I try to hold my breath: one, two, three, four . . . I count inside my head, trying to see if I can reach 100. Maybe if I do my father will think me dead, and leave me alone.

I am scared, so scared. I feel rough hands scrabbling at my thighs, and then he has his fingers inside me. It hurts. It always hurts so much. He shifts his weight, and pushes his flesh into my hand. He's breathing heavily now, and laughing to himself. I smell his smell. Stale sweat mixed with the sweet, sickly scent of the coconut oil he uses in his hair.

It sickens me. I feel so dirty and so ashamed.

73

Then my father rapes me. He does so repeatedly. I do not want to live. I want to die. I want death to come as a cold embrace that will end all my father's predatory, vicious, sadistic ones.

I can't let him see me cry. I can't let him see my pain, or hear my pain. I can't let him see how much it hurts me, and how much it destroys me inside. My father would love that. He would love to see my terror and my pain and my sick, shameful hurt.

To him, it would show that his 'punishment' is working.

Whenever I emerged form the horrors of the cellar I felt so dirty and defiled. I would hang my head in shame and try not to meet my mother's eye. She in turn would try to bury herself in her work, clanging pans at the stove. It was her way of pretending that I wasn't there – a tired, dishevelled little girl with crumpled, bloodied clothing, standing at the top of those dark and hateful steps.

A little girl rank with sex and violence. A daughter whose father had spent the last two days punishing her – by raping and beating her.

'Can I go shower?' I'd mumble, eventually.

I felt as if I should say sorry to Mum somehow – sorry for letting him do this to me. Sorry for not being good enough. Sorry for having done bad, and making Dad punish me again. I felt as if Mum must blame me and be angry with me. But I could never find the right words to say that I was sorry. So, like Mum, I just tried to ignore what had happened, to bury it deep. I tried to act like normal. What else was I to do?

'Can I go shower?' I'd say.

'If you need to,' Mum would reply, without turning to look at me.

I'd turn away from her narrow, hunched back, and head for the stairs and the bathroom. As I did, I would imagine that I'd see my mother's shoulders shaking and trembling, shuddering and wracked with sobs. I'd imagine that really, she did care and that she was mortified for me. Should I go check on Mum, I'd wonder. Should I go ask if she was okay? Had my bad, dirty behaviour with Dad in the cellar really made her that sad? I was torn apart by guilt and shame. Guilt and shame.

But perhaps I was imagining it all? Perhaps if I went to 'comfort' Mum, she'd just turn on me?

As for Dad, he just didn't seem to give a damn. He'd emerge from raping me, violently, in the cellar, and change his shalwar kamiz for a fresh white one – no doubt washed and perfectly ironed by Mum and me – and head off down to the mosque. Maybe he thought his god could absolve his sins.

But sins like those, sins like those he visited on me – they could never be forgiven, not in a million years.

When my father was abusing me, my brothers were often at home – but they spent their time watching football on TV, or intheir rooms listening to music. As soon as they were old enough they got out of the house – taking weekend jobs in the newsagents, or other shops in town. And when they weren't working they would hang out with their friends. I was not allowed to do any of these things. I had to stay at home with Mum, doing the chores and waiting on the men of the house. Or at least that's what I did when I wasn't being abused by Dad.

Sometimes, I did risk complaining to my lazy, pampered brothers.

'I'm not your slave,' I'd tell them. 'Go and do it yourself! You've got hands and feet, haven't you!'

Billy would try to talk me around. 'But I'm tired, Hannan, please . . .'

But Zakir and Raz would get angry if I didn't do exactly as they said, and they would threaten to tell Dad. Whenever they made that threat, I caved in right away. Dad would blow a fuse if I disobeyed any of his sons, with the threat of 'punishment' never far away. Occasionally, Billy did try to clear the plates from the table, or even to wash up. And he used to try to speak to Mum and me in a gentle, kindly way.

'Come on, Mum, you can't do the hoovering *again*,' he'd tell her. 'Here, let me have a go.'

Mum would try to object. She didn't want Billy helping. She knew the rules of the house. But sometimes, Billy would insist, and Mum would be too tired to resist him. If Dad found out he would blow his top at Billy, scolding him for doing 'women's work'. He hated any of the boys breaking the rules, just as he did with me.

My father encouraged the boys to do what he thought was work fitting for a man: making the call to prayer on the loud-speaker system at the mosque.

Allah is most Great (repeated four times)
I bear witness that there is no other god but Allah (repeated
    two times)
I bear witness that Mohammed is the messenger of Allah
    (repeated two times)
Come to Prayer (repeated two times)
Come to Success (repeated two times)
Allah is most great (repeated twice)
There is no god but Allah

But Billy hated doing the call to prayer, and he refused to be totally cowed by my father. Whenever we had visitors, the men would sit in the front room with the women serving them. Billy would try to remain with the women. He would be in the kitchen, talking to Mum and me as we worked, and trying to lend a hand. Dad found this deeply insulting, for it 'showed him up' in front of his men friends.

With three brothers and my father to wait on hand and foot, the daily chores were never-ending. My least favourite job was washing the clothes. We hand-washed everything in the kitchen sink, because we didn't have a washing machine. Mum used a big bar of green soap to lather up the dirty clothes, before rinsing them. And she would bleach the whites until they were white as snow.

My job was to carry the baskets of washing in and out and help fold the big sheets. I had to hide all the female underwear – the bras and panties – so that the men of the house couldn't see them. My brothers didn't care one way or the other, but Dad would fly into a rage if any women's underwear was visible. Of course, it was fine for us to see his dirty underwear, or my brothers', for we had to wash it all by hand. But I had to hang our undies to dry in our bedroom, out of the view of my father.

Over time I learned well the harsh routine of my chores. On a school day I would be the first to get up. I would wake around seven, go downstairs, and make traditional Pakistani tea. Then I'd do heaps of toast under the grill, and butter it. I would take the tea and toast into the back lounge, and open a packet of custard cream biscuits and arrange them on a plate.

I'd eat my breakfast on my own, before everyone else woke up. After that, I'd take up my position by the sink, doing the washing up from the night before. Then I'd rush around getting myself ready for school. Once Sabina was old enough, I also had to get her out of bed and help her dress. Finally, we'd head off to school with Mum as our escort.

We took packed lunches that Mum had prepared the night before – jam sandwiches, and an apple or a banana. I knew the other kids would have all sorts of fancy things in their lunch boxes, but I didn't mind. I really liked jam sandwiches. My favourite was Morrisons' own brand strawberry jam on white bread, with the crusts left on. It was a good thing I liked it, because that was what I always got!

I didn't need to be ordered to do my chores any more. The threat of the abuse had made me easy to control, which in turn made Mum's life easier. Once I knew I was expected to do something, I just did it. Anything to avoid the cellar. Even my little sister, Sabina, started treating me as someone to be ordered about. She'd seen the way the others behaved, and followed their lead. If I asked her to help me taking things through to the kitchen, she mostly refused.

At the end of the school day Mum would walk us home in time for our Quran lesson. Once that was over I would be allowed sit and watch television with tea and biscuits. After that I had to rush through my homework, and then start helping with the evening meal. We ate dinner at about eight, and then I'd help clear up until it was time for bed. I used to try to get to bed early, for I knew I had to be up early the next morning.

Saturday was laundry day, which I dreaded. By the evening I'd be exhausted, and I would retreat to my bed to read a library book by the light of the single bulb. Whenever I had the chance I would have my nose stuck in a book. As with my world of make-believe, reading was a way to escape from reality. I used to re-read books that our teachers had read to us at school, because doing so reminded me of happy times – my school days. Having an adult dedicate time to read to me was a sign of real affection, and an absolute treat. I wanted to relive those moments as much as I could.

One of my most-loved books was called *Flat Stanley*, about a boy who gets accidentally flattened and then has all sorts of new and magical abilities as a flat person. But my absolute favourite were the *Please Mrs Butler* poems, the best of which was called 'A dog in the playground'. It went like this:

> *Dog in the playground,*
> *Suddenly there.*
> *Smile on his face,*
> *Tail in the air.*
>
> *Dog in the playground,*
> *Bit of a fuss:*
> *I know that dog –*
> *Lives next to us!*
>
> *Dog in the playground:*
> *Oh no he don't.*
> *He'll come with me,*
> *You'll see if he won't.*
>
> *The word gets round;*
> *The crowd gets bigger.*
> *His name's Bob.*
> *It ain't – it's Trigger.*

And so it went. I loved the Mrs Butler poems in part because they were so realistic. They were written in the way that we would talk to each other at school. They spoke of life on the streets of my hometown, if not quite the reality of life on my street.

Once every two months Mum would take us to the library in the town centre. We were each allowed to choose five books to take home. I started reading the Judy Blume books, which are all about girls growing up. The way they were written made me laugh. I loved the character called Fudge, a real tomboy-type. She didn't like what other girls liked – gossiping and girly stuff. And she was a bit of a loner, just like me.

Fudge's life was set in the USA, and the books told of her relationship with her eccentric American parents. Her comments about her family were so funny. There were lots of Americanisms in there: she called her mother 'Mom', and her class was called 'First Grade'. And, later, she had secret crushes on boys at school. To me Fudge's life seemed so adventurous and exotic.

Despite my love of reading I had no books of my own, and there were precious few in the house. Other than the Quran, Dad would read a Pakistani newspaper, The Daily Jang, which the newsagent got in every Friday. He read all the Pakistani news, plus the cricket results. And then there were a handful of books on Islam, and Pakistani history, in the house.

Although Dad wasn't physically living in Pakistan, in his mind he was still back in the village. In his day-to-day he tried to avoid anything that might shatter the illusion of his Pakistani existence, and bring home to him that he was living in a town in the north of England. He never read anything about England – whether newspapers, magazines, or books – and tried to maintain a strict insularity.

After Saturday's laundry, Sunday was ironing day. I would spend the day in the bedroom, ironing the clothes for our family of eight, whilst Mum was downstairs cooking and cleaning. The boys' shirts were the most difficult to do, with their fiddly collars. I could never get all the creases out, and each one would take ages. But at least left alone with the ironing I could retreat into my daydreams.

I'd listen to the chart show on a little transistor radio that we had in the bedroom. I'd gaze out over the terraces, my mind lost in a dream. Gradually, the neatly ironed clothes would pile up on the bed. When I was done ironing I had to sort the clothes out, and put them away neatly on the right shelves – ours in our room; the boys' in their rooms; my hated father's in his room.

I knew that I had to be especially careful when it came to Dad's clothes. If I ironed them 'badly', or put them back on his shelves 'the wrong way', it was an excuse for him to 'punish' me. All the time I worked this threat was in the back of my mind, hanging over me like a dark and evil cloud.

As time went on it became more and more common for me to wake alone on the cold cellar floor. The rest of the family responded by treating it as if it was somehow normal to have me locked in the cellar. If it was a school day, Mum would have to get up early and make the breakfast instead of me. If it was a weekend and I missed my chores, I would have to do the ironing in the week after school.

It was no secret to anyone in the family that I was being 'punished' and imprisoned. They all simply accepted it as another of Dad's 'rules'.

School holidays were the very worst times. At least school gifted me a few hours when I didn't have to worry about Dad. But during the holidays there was no escape. For weeks on end I had to stay in the house doing all the chores, and being ordered around by the males. Sabina was rarely made to help, and I felt like a slave. I felt like everyone's slave. And if I 'messed up', Dad would haul me off for 'punishment'.

Any excuse was good enough for him to visit his evil, abusive ways on me. And Dad was like a terrifying predator. I never knew when he would strike. Once I was in the bathroom, when all of a sudden Dad just barged in. He locked the door, and ordered me to remain exactly where I was, standing at the sink, but to turn and face him. The bathroom was horribly cramped, so I was basically right next to him.

He took down his shalwar kamiz baggy pants, and plunked

himself down on the loo. He forced me to watch as he started touching himself and breathing heavily. I tried to look away, in disgust, but he grabbed me by the hair and forced my face towards him – so close that I could smell that horrible, musty smell that always made me feel so sick. Then he grabbed my hand and forced it around his flesh.

It was disgusting, him forcing me to do this right there in that claustrophobic, smelly toilet. I wanted to vomit. I wanted to run and get out of there, and I tried to struggle, but he tore at my hair more savagely, forcing me back towards him. The more I struggled and he hurt me, the more he enjoyed it. That, I knew well by now, was how my father really got his kicks.

Irrational thought filled my head. I wanted to die, and yet at the same time I was afraid my father might kill me. With a grunt he was done. He stopped, and pulled up his baggy pants. He elbowed me out of the way and went to wash at the sink.

'Remember, I'll kill you if you ever breathe a word,' he hissed, his eyes cold and dark pits of loathing. 'You're dirty and worthless and you're going to hell. It's all a cursed, evil *girl* like you deserves.'

He shut the door on me, his feet clumping off down the stairs. I slumped over the washbasin and vomited my guts up, retching and retching until there was nothing left but bitter bile. But still the dirty, disgusting smell of him lingered on me. I would never be clean.

Dad never once let me forget that he had never wanted a girl child. But I knew that the abuse was also triggered by my rebellious ways, and by my standing up to him. In an effort to protect Mum I had put myself in the firing line. My rebellion had triggered his anger, and tipped it over into full violence. He had decided that I was a disrespectful, cursed daughter, and that I needed to be beaten into submission. From there, it was just a short step to unleashing his sexual violence on me.

After a year or two of the abuse, even Mum would turn on me, telling me how 'worthless' and 'useless' I was. My father's sickness seemed to have infected the whole family. I knew that other firstborn girls on my street were also made to help in the home. But they seemed so much freer and happier than me, with barely a fraction of the workload. And I couldn't imagine any of them being so horribly abused.

But if they had been, I suppose it was unlikely that anyone in our community would have realised.

As a family we survived on donations to the mosque, and on the generosity of the British taxpayer. Dad was on income support and we were on housing benefit. Dad had managed to claim the dole by lying to the council. He had claimed to be unemployed, but of course he wasn't. Dad was the community's full-time Imam, and he did get paid, from the cash donations to the mosque.

Lying to get benefits wasn't seen as being dishonourable in our community, although being caught by the authorities and outed for doing so would be. Honour wasn't so much about what you did. It was about what you were seen to be doing, or caught doing publicly. A lot of people in our community had a public and a private face, and that was how they maintained their 'honour'.

Indeed, in my father's mind he may have seen nothing wrong in locking his infant daughter in the cellar and beating and raping her. As long as no one knew about it publicly, it would attract no 'dishonour' to the family or the community, and neither would it besmirch his good name as the community Imam. Therefore, how could it be 'dishonourable'?

Likewise, while everyone in the community knew Dad was on income support whilst serving as their full-time Imam, no one thought that was *wrong*. Only if he got caught did it become an issue. Even then Dad might well have argued that taking what you could from the land of immorality and disbelief was fair game. And who in the community would have gone against him? No one. Dad was in an unassailable position as the Imam, especially as the mosque committee was made up of his friends.

When I was growing up I didn't think that Dad was doing something wrong, either. I knew that he was on income support, and I knew that we got council benefits. I knew that he worked as the Imam, and received donations for doing so. But I didn't think that any of this was wrong, for no one in the community ever so much as questioned it. I just concluded that that was how Imams, and their families, got by.

Whenever we had mail we would have to open it and tell Dad what it was. He barely read a word of English. If it was a bill, then we'd tell him the amount to pay, and fill in the pay slip. He'd sign a cheque, and take it down to the post office. And if it was a dole form we'd fill it in to his instructions, and show him where to sign.

The housing benefit came automatically, on the basis of my parents being on the dole. And once a week Dad had to go to the Job Centre and sign, to show that he was 'available' for work. Of course, he never intended to get a job. He acted as if he was somehow above it all, because he was an Imam: his religious calling came above the normal responsibilities of a citizen and a father.

Yet every single aspect of my father's life – the food he ate; the heating that warmed his home; his children's education and their healthcare; the very water he drank – all of it was funded by the British state. And it was that same British state that he in turn abhorred, and attempted to ensure that his children abhorred – by bringing them up with the same attitudes and blind prejudices that he had.

It was only my father who seemed to believe that he had a God-given right to avoid 'normal' responsibilities. Other men in the street worked and paid their taxes. Some of them had their own businesses. The father of one of my friends ran a halal dairy farm, and he sold eggs and milk to shops around town. Amina's dad, Abdul, was a hard-working bus driver. There were other men on our street who didn't work, but it was invariably for good reasons – like ill-health.

Fortunately, my brothers didn't follow in my father's ways. They studied and worked hard. In fact, Zakir turned out to be a bit of an entrepreneur. When he was just twelve a local Indian shopkeeper gave him a job as a paperboy, and he soon graduated to working behind the counter. The shopkeeper was a Hindu, but he could tell that Zakir was a talented salesman. Zakir was saving up money for university, and so he needed every penny he could earn.

Sponging off the state wasn't a tradition, either. People worked hard back in the village in Pakistan. It was unique to my father, because he was the Imam. He believed he was only supposed to concern himself with matters of the spirit. He was supposed to be above and immune to earthly worries or law. Others somehow accepted that, because they saw him as focusing on the 'spiritual health' of the community.

Nobody would ever have dreamt of reporting Dad for being on the dole. In a sense, he was above reproach. This immunity from criticism spilled over into everything he did. Dad saw his status as a holy man justifying whatever he chose to do: lying to the government; stealing from the state; beating Mum and me; even raping his own daughter. Everything was justifiable in my father's mind.

By the time I was ten I had learned to read the entire Quran, which is some six hundred pages long. Most children didn't manage this until they were much older. Normally, parents would have a big celebration, throwing a party and handing out sweets to the whole community. But in my case absolutely nothing happened.

I had struggled to achieve this largely to please my parents. Part of me still hoped to win Dad's recognition and his affection. I longed to prove to him I wasn't a cursed, worthless, evil girl. *See, Dad, I'm good, I'm good – I can read the entire Quran!* But my father's reaction was simply to ignore it. It was as if nothing had happened.

I felt devastated. I could do nothing right in his eyes.

Chapter Eight

A Caged Bird Crying

I approached the age of eleven and it was time for me to prepare for secondary school. My final primary school report gave me a mix of B and C grades, which wasn't too bad. Billy read the report to Mum, going through it subject by subject. Mum actually congratulated me, saying how well I'd done 'for a girl'. But Dad ignored it. I wasn't surprised. By now it was what I expected. At least ignoring it was neutral.

Still, I did feel pleased with my results. They weren't exceptional, but between the domestic drudgery and the nightmare of the abuse, it was a wonder that I had done even this well. My brothers had done a lot better than me, but they'd been given every opportunity to do so.

My parents wanted me to go to a Muslim girls' school. This wasn't because they cared about my education – it was all about 'honour'. The Muslim girls' school was thought to be 'safe', and insulated from the evils of British society – like smoking, drinking and boys. Dad believed that mainstream secondary schools were dens of iniquity and sin. But the Muslim girls' school was fee-paying, and the reason I didn't end up going there was because my parents couldn't afford it.

I was glad they couldn't afford to send me. It was the last sort of school that I wanted to attend. I was starting to associate my religion – Islam – with submission, pain and suffering. To me a Muslim school meant more of the same.

My brothers were going to a fine school just outside of town. It took them an hour to get there every morning by bus, and an hour back again. But my parents couldn't be bothered to send me there. There was also a grammar school, but you had to sit an entrance exam to get in. There was no suggestion that I might do so, as no one thought me very intelligent.

And so, by default I ended up going to the local comprehensive, commonly known as 'Bermford Comp'. It was famous for being the worst school in town. Its pupils came from the local area, which was working-class and poverty-ridden. There was a lot of crime in the area, and a good number of the local families were in trouble with the police.

Sadly, Jane and Susan went to the Bishop Tate School, a state-run establishment, but one with a far better reputation than Bermford Comp. My parents wouldn't even consider sending me there, because you had to be a practising Catholic in order to get in. Jane and Susan made sure they went to church just a few times before they applied, to justify doing so. Then they moved house, to be nearer the school, and that was the last contact I ever had with them.

My junior school had been Church of England, but it hadn't seemed much of an issue for my parents back then. Every year I had gone to Bermford Parish Church, for Easter and Christmas outings. We used to go around the church grounds doing rubbings of gravestones and brass plaques. There was one plaque I remember commemorating the man who had invented a machine for turning wool into yarn. We learned all about it in our lessons on local history.

But now that I was almost eleven years old – and approaching marriageable age in the rural Pakistani mindset – Dad wanted control over my schooling. Back in the village, girls were often married off by the time they were eleven. And God knows what my father might have in mind for me, now that I had reached that age.

In fact, Dad was becoming increasingly more authoritarian with all of his daughters. By now my little sister, Aliya, was going to the same Church of England junior school that I had attended. Being a talkative type, she would come home telling stories about the vicar, and all the exciting things he had told them about Jesus and Christianity. That was enough! Dad didn't shout at her as he had me, but he was enraged that little Aliya was being exposed to all this *Christianity*.

Dad alerted the community to the 'danger' of their children being 'indoctrinated' in this way. And the parents in turn complained to the school. Faced with such a groundswell of opposition, the school authorities relented in part. From then on, Muslim children were allowed to stay in the classroom and given some colouring to do during church visits. It was another 'victory' for the blind prejudice of my father.

I quickly made new friends at Bermford Comp – including Amanda, Karen, Lara, and Iram. Iram was a Pakistani Muslim girl, and my only Muslim friend at school. She lived the other side of town from us. Karen was striking-looking, with red hair, a petite stature and snowy white skin. As for Amanda, she was very beautiful, with lustrous brown hair and deep hazel eyes. But it was my English friend Lara who was the real belle of the bunch. She was tall, with coal-dark hair cut boyishly short, and smouldering, laughter-filled eyes. All the boys fancied Lara.

From the start, Lara was my best friend and my protector. Under her influence, the other girls did their best to make me feel like one of them. But I could never quite forget that I was an outsider. Karen's father made it horribly clear that he didn't want me to be friends with his daughter. One day we were waiting at the bus stop outside the school gates when a car pulled up. A man wound down the window and started yelling at Karen.

'Get in the car! Just get in! What're you doing standing there talking to that bloody Paki?'

Karen didn't know what to say, or where to look. She said a rushed goodbye, and jumped into her father's car. Away it squealed with a screech of angry tyres.

When I saw her the next day she looked mortified. Karen was a good friend and I didn't want to make it an issue. Both of us must have decided not to mention it, for we never did. We just remained friends anyway. But from then on she wouldn't wait with me at the school gates.

And so I learned that the racism didn't just go the one way. I knew that my dad hated white people, and here it seemed was a white person who hated me. But why was it always the adults causing such blind hatred, whilst we children did our best to get along? The race issue came to a head one day, and in the most horrible of ways.

My school friend Amanda seemed to me to be the girl who had everything: beauty, a great personality, and a lovely family. Her house was near the school, and sometimes we'd go there for lunch. Her father was a businessman and her mother was a housewife. Her mum was really nice, and lucky old Amanda seemed able to tell her mum anything. What was more, Amanda told me how her father looked after and supported her.

I would have given anything to have Amanda's life. It wasn't her good looks I coveted. I wasn't bothered about being popular with the boys. Even though she was beautiful, that wasn't what I envied. I just wanted the love and stability of a normal healthy family. I would have given up my own parents in a flash, had Amanda's offered me a home.

Towards the end of that first term I arranged to meet Amanda in the town centre. It was lunchtime on a Saturday, a time when I knew Dad would be at the mosque. Feeling brave, I invited Amanda to my house to hang out. I had been to her place so many times, it seemed rude not to. Yet I had never in my life invited a friend into my home. I knew it was risky, and I was nervous. I wasn't worried about Mum. She wouldn't really mind. My fear was all about Dad.

The front door was always unlocked, so we walked right in. I took Amanda into the lounge. We sat on the sofa and started talking. Mum brought us a drink and some biscuits, and I began to relax a little. Maybe it was all going to be okay. But all of a sudden there was the click of the front door latch, and without warning in walked my father. For whatever reason he had chosen this day of all days to come home early.

I froze stiff as he caught sight of Amanda. An instant later he was standing at the open door, ordering me out of the room. I knew what was coming. He closed the door roughly behind me and started yelling at me in Punjabi.

'How dare you bring that gori here! In my house! How many times do I have to tell you? They're dirty infidels. They sleep around! They have no belief . . .'

On and on he ranted. It wasn't as if I hadn't heard this a thousand times before.

'I don't want her in my house!' he shouted. 'And I won't have you having gori friends!'

When Dad started ranting there was no point in even chancing a reply. I just hung my head and hoped Amanda wouldn't realise what he was saying. Suddenly, he was done and he stalked off into the men's lounge. At least there was no dragging me into the cellar with Amanda sitting there waiting.

I went back into the lounge, burning up with shame and embarrassment. I felt so bad at what I had done to my friend. I had invited Amanda in, knowing how my Dad would react if he caught us.

'I'm really sorry,' I muttered. 'Dad says I have to go and pray. Is it okay if you leave now?'

'Of course,' said Amanda. She jumped up and gave me a big hug. Even though I was trying to hide it she could see how upset I was. 'Don't worry. Enjoy your prayers, and I'll see you at school.'

After that Dad knew that I would never dare bring anyone else home. If he went off like that again in front of one of my friends, I would simply die of the shame.

On the Monday I was at school sitting next to Amanda. I apologised for having to make her leave so soon. I tried explaining to her that Dad didn't like English people, because he didn't understand them. It was the best excuse that I could think of.

Amanda gave a knowing smile. 'I thought he had some sort of issue with me. He did seem very angry . . . I hope I didn't cause you any trouble. But we were having such a nice time, weren't we? Pity he had to go and spoil it.'

'It's not you,' I tried to say. 'Really it's not. So please, don't feel bad about it. It's my dad's problem, not yours. In fact, he is the problem!'

But no matter what we said I still felt bad about it. I'd been to her house, and her parents had been so lovely to me – and this is how my father treated her. Why did I always have to be the weirdo, with the nasty, unwelcoming family?

I wanted to tell my friends as much of the truth as I could, because I wanted them to know where I was coming from. I wanted them to understand that I came from a place that was so different from theirs, and that's why things sometimes seemed so odd in my life. I wanted them to know that the hatred and the hostility didn't come from me.

But I couldn't just say to Amanda that my dad hated white people and was a racist. That was such an ugly word. It would hurt me to say it, and it could hurt Amanda. I didn't want her to feel like she was dirty or worthless, because she most definitely wasn't. I was using my culture as a smoke screen to hide Dad's faults, and to save Amanda's feelings.

And of course, Amanda had only seen the very tip of the iceberg. She had no idea how truly dark and abusive was my life at home with my father.

At secondary school all the girls had to wear a navy blue skirt and white shirt, plus a navy blazer. My skirt fell just below my knees, but that wasn't enough for my father. Beneath it I had to wear navy cotton trousers – shalwar kamiz style. I hated having to do so. Once again, I was destined to be the odd-one-out.

'Why do you have those weird trousers on?' one of the other pupils asked.

I shrugged, resignedly. 'I'm not allowed to show my legs.' It sounded such a stupid thing to say.

'Not allowed to show your legs! Why not? What's wrong with them?'

'Nothing,' I'd mutter. 'It's because of my religion.'

At that I'd get the strangest of looks, and it would usually be the end of the conversation. Religion wasn't our main top topic of conversation at secondary school!

I was approaching the age of puberty now, and this was in part what drove my father's paranoia. When a Muslim girl from our community starts her period, she is barred from the mosque, she isn't allowed to touch the Quran, or even to pray at home. The Quran says quite clearly that menstruation is an 'indisposition', and that menstruating women are 'unclean'.

Puberty meant that there were a lot of new taboo subjects at home. Mum had never told me that I would start my period at some point. It was taboo. Even the stuff that I had seen at school, during sex education lessons, didn't tell me how to deal with it, or where to get tampons or towels. So when my period did start it was all very scary. Fortunately, I was at school at the time and I went straight to the nurse. She explained everything to me, and gave me a few packs of free sanitary towels.

I was the first amongst my school friends to start my period. They were keen to know just how it felt. This gave me a brief spell of unexpected popularity! Amongst my girlfriends it made me somehow special. But at home it was very different. Because menstruating women are seen as 'unclean', I associated my own menstruation with sin and dirt. I didn't tell Mum for months on end. But eventually I ran out of sanitary towels, so I had to confess to her what was happening.

She told me that I was not to use tampons, because putting something unnatural into your body was considered 'wrong' in Islam. She told me that I couldn't pray when I had my period, which was a great excuse as far as I was concerned to avoid my religious 'duties', and to stay away from the mosque completely. Every cloud had a silver lining.

As for Dad, he didn't realise that I had started menstruating for a year or more. He was used to me bleeding whenever he sexually assaulted me, so at first he didn't notice. But once he had realised he avoided raping me at those times, for I was too 'unclean' for him to go near me. Other girls at school moaned about their periods, and the pain of being 'on'. But for me it was a blessed release.

During that first year at secondary school, Dad was abusing me as often as before. At least once a month he'd drag me into the cellar and rape me. But I had a new, more mature group of friends now, and they started to notice my bruising. It must have been obvious that all wasn't right, especially when we changed for PE. I'd have bruising around my breasts, where he'd been groping me, and around my thighs. But no one ever challenged me to explain it, and I had no desire to reveal all.

As the abuse continued, I started to think about escape. The only way out I could see was to get away to college or university, or to kill myself. I considered running away from home, but the only people I knew well in my home town were Muslims, and they would take me back to my father, because he was their Imam. There was no way on earth that I could tell them what was happening. They just wouldn't believe that such a thing was possible.

I felt burdened with shame the whole time. I felt disgusting and dirty. Part of me felt evil, as if I deserved what he did to me. I had been brainwashed by Dad into believing what he told me. I felt that I deserved it, because he told me that I deserved it. I deserved it for being evil and unworthy of his God. I was trapped in the vicious circle of the brainwashing and the abuse. If Dad had been doing this to my sisters, I would have known straight away that it was wrong. But not when he was doing it to me.

I lived for the promise of escape. It was the promise of escape that drove my hopes to do well at secondary school. If I studied hard I might win a place to go to Sixth Form College, or university. I knew of girls in our community who had left home to do further studies. I knew that would give me a way out, for then Dad would have no access to me. It was the only sure route of escape that I could see.

But I was far from sure if my parents would ever let me go. I just knew that girls from our street had got away to college, finding freedom when they did so. That was my longed-for route of escape. But I was only an eleven-year-old girl, and college was at least six years away.

That summer I was overjoyed when my father decided to spend the holidays back in the village in Pakistan. For me, it meant several weeks of blessed release. But it meant something very different for my brother Raz. Raz was sixteen years old, and my father took him with him 'on holiday' to Pakistan. I just presumed that Raz would return at the end of the holidays, and start Sixth Form College.

But when Dad returned there was no Raz. I asked Billy where he might be. Raz was in a madrassa – a Quranic school – Billy explained, starting his training to be a *hafiz* – someone who has learned the Quran off by heart. After three years, Raz would be able to quote any verse of it in Arabic from memory alone.

I didn't know anything about what a Pakistani madrassa might be like. But it seemed to me that Dad had made Raz stay there to do what he wanted him to. There had certainly been no mention of this before they left, nor any special goodbyes. Like many things in our household, it was all down to Dad's will.

People used to say of Raz that he was the 'dunce' of the boys in our family. A girl's level of intelligence didn't really warrant comment – only her 'honour' and her looks. But I thought Raz a gentle, simple soul. I was sad to see him go, and I worried for him. I wondered how he might be faring in that distant land where Dad had sent him.

My own Quran studies had been so hateful, and I couldn't imagine what it would be like to be forced to learn the entire thing by rote, especially in an alien language. From the beating that I'd experienced myself in the mosque, I couldn't imagine that this Pakistani madrassa would be a benign learning environment. In fact, in my mind it was a place of brutality and violence. I just hoped that sensitive Raz would pull though all right.

There were one or two people in our community who were

hafiz of the Quran. They were the ones who would do the Quran reading at special times, like Ramadan. They could do so without even having the book in front of them. It was a mark of great status in our community – status that my father, the Imam, no doubt coveted. It was via poor Raz that he aimed to achieve this new 'honour' – having a hafiz in the family.

I wasn't to see Raz again for another three years.

That first year at secondary school I joined the netball, hockey and athletics teams. In athletics I ran for the school – long-distance and cross-country. The schools in our area had a league for each of these sports. Bermford Comp may not have been very academically inclined, but it did excel at sports. Hockey was my favourite game, and our school was top of the league for two years running.

My main positions were left back or goalkeeper. I may not have been very big in stature, but I was fearless. I used to love bashing the ball really hard, and clearing the girls from the opposing team out of the way! The hockey pitch was my place to work out all my pent-up aggression, and my internalised pain. Having so often faced my dad's raging violence, there was little that I could see to fear on the hockey field.

I loved being part of a team, especially as Lara played in the hockey squad alongside me. We were all there doing our bit, and we had to work together to win. Because we were on a winning streak, there was a lot of laughter and celebrations. It felt great to be in a team and doing well. I came right out of myself when playing hockey.

But one day I was in the showers after a hockey match when the inevitable happened: Lara noticed that my chest was covered in bruises. She reached out her hand in involuntary alarm, then drew it back to her face in horror. Her eyes met mine, wide with concern. She gestured at the nasty black and blue bruising.

'What happened?' she gasped. 'Surely that's not from the hockey . . .'

I shook my head. We did get knocked about a bit, but mainly on our shins.

'So how did . . . Did someone . . . I mean, who did it to you?'

'I fell down,' I lied. I reached for the soap, hiding my eyes from Lara as I did so. 'I fell, that's all.'

'How did you fall and only hurt your boobs?' Lara queried. I could tell she was worried for me.

I shrugged. 'I dunno. I just fell down the stairs.'

Lara stared at me for a few seconds, and then she must have decided to let it be. I felt so dirty. I scrubbed at my skin with the soap, imagining that I could smell my father on me. But no matter how hard I scrubbed, I couldn't get clean. I had lied to my best friend. I couldn't bring myself to tell her that the bruises marked where my father had been groping my chest, as he locked me in the shadow of the nightmare and raped me.

As I peddled those lies, and saw the doubt in Lara's eyes, I felt like a fraud and a betrayer. And it was then that I realised that my body, and my life, were no longer my own. Dad owned my body. He could do whatever he liked with it. And I had no control over it whatsoever. I was just something to be used.

My friends at school were nearly all white, for there were few Asian pupils. There was so much about those white kids' lives that I envied. All the love and kindness that they received from their parents. All the adventures they went on as a family. All the freedom they had to be children and to grow.

By contrast, my life was hellish, and full of shameful dirt and darkness. My childhood had been ripped apart by my father. Part of me still believed that I deserved to be punished, although I could never understand exactly what I had done wrong. Part of me believed it when he told me I was going straight to hell.

Riven by self-disgust and doubt, I became more bitter and angry and introverted. Not surprisingly, real trouble lay ahead.

Chapter Nine

Rebellion's Spring

I still read my Quran most days before I went to sleep. I didn't understand the Arabic words, but I had been told so often that simply saying them was a virtuous act. Part of me was still trying to become 'good' – to earn my way into my father's affections. At the same time Dad was still using his 'religion' to justify his behaviour. I was still 'evil', and I deserved my 'punishment' as the only way to 'cure' me.

When I read the Quran I prayed for my life to get better, but it never did. So I began praying for my father to die, instead. I knew that doing so was 'sinful', but I couldn't help it. If he died, I reasoned, then he couldn't abuse me any more. I knew that the rest of the family treated me like a domestic slave in part because they followed his example. Everything that was painful in my life flowed from him. If he was dead, it was bound to get better.

So I prayed to Allah to take Dad's life away. I didn't really think it would happen, but it helped me deal with my anger. In any case, my prayers were never answered. And over time I began to think that God – *my father's god* – wasn't listening. I began to think that my father's god was a cruel and avenging one, with no room for love or happiness in his heart. Increasingly, I saw Allah in the image of my father.

In my mind, God seemed more inclined to condemn people and laugh at their misfortunes. He certainly did nothing to alleviate my own misery. He threw people into the fires of hell, and had them hung up by their hair – or at least that's what my father said. I believed that hell was a pit full of eternal fire, one that was constantly filling up with people who had done wrong – evil sinners like me. I lived in fear of God, my mother and my father.

By contrast, when I went to visit my school friends I was amazed to hear how they chatted away happily with their parents. They talked about their weekends, about meeting their mates in town, and about going shopping together. They even talked about the boys they liked, and who was going out with whom. If I was lucky, I would have spent my weekend chained to the kitchen sink, scrubbing dishes. Or I might have spent it hand-washing the clothes of a household of eight, and doing all the ironing.

Or, if I had been really unfortunate, I would have been locked in the darkness of the cellar, being 'punished' by my father.

By now I was twelve and I had made a new best friend on our street. Everyone knew her by her nickname – 'Skip'. Skip was five years my senior and she was a Muslim of Pakistani parentage. I admired Skip because of her courage, honesty and self-confidence. Plus, she was a real tomboy and very funny with it.

Skip was a born rebel. She and I would spend our time booting around a football in her back yard, and laughing happily. But if Dad caught me playing football he'd fly into a rage. Playing football was 'shameful', he'd rant, and not for good Muslim girls. We should be inside, cooking and cleaning for the menfolk. Once Dad was gone, Skip would roll her eyes and make fun of him. To her, Dad was a throwback to a dark past.

Skip was seventeen years old, and she felt she was quite able to handle herself. But I felt as if I had a split personality. At school, I was a totally different person than I was at home. I never, ever talked to my school friends about my home life. But, when I was with Skip, I realised that I wasn't alone in facing such problems. Skip wasn't getting abused by her father, of that I'm certain, but she did share any number of other fears with me.

Skip's greatest worry was that her father was going to force her into an arranged marriage. He was more of a businessman than a man of religion, but that didn't mean that he didn't want an arranged marriage for his daughter. This wasn't about religion –

it was all about culture and tradition. And, of course, it was about 'honour'.

Skip and I were forever discussing the forced marriages that other girls in the street had suffered. Skip was the sort of girl who wouldn't be forced into anything. She wanted to fall in love, and marry for love. We used to fantasise about finding the perfect man and about the perfect wedding. Skip and I shared a dream of getting an education – her to free herself from the control of the 'community', me to free myself from the darkness of home. And we fantasised about finding love.

Skip was a true free spirit. She was the only girl on our street who I felt was similar to me. Towards the end of the first year of our friendship, Skip told me she was going on holiday to Pakistan. She wasn't unduly worried. She'd been to the village several times before with her parents. There hadn't been the slightest hint that an arranged marriage might be in the offing. Her father was far too civilised to spring one on her.

Two days after Skip had left for Pakistan there was a phone call at home. My mum answered and it turned out that it was Skip. It wasn't unusual for her to call me, but why was she doing so from Pakistan? I sensed trouble.

I took the phone from Mum. 'Hi, Skip, how are . . .'

'Hannan? Hannan? Thank God you're there,' Skip cut in, her voice crackling with tension and fear. 'Listen, I need your help. I've got to be quick. If they catch me on the phone . . .'

Skip proceeded to tell me how she had been taken to visit some distant relatives somewhere in the northeast of Pakistan. Upon arrival at the village she had been presented with a Pakistani man – a 'cousin' whom she'd never even met before. Out of the blue she was told that this was the man she was going to marry.

Skip had been locked alone in a dark room with no food or water until she 'agreed' to go through with the marriage. Rather than starve or die of thirst, she had done so. But somehow she managed to get to a phone and was calling me out of sheer desperation. She was determined to escape. She asked me to speak to her older sister, Saira, and get help. Most of all, she needed a flight out of Pakistan.

I felt so sorry for Skip, but part of me wasn't exactly surprised. How many other girls did we know that this had happened to? Dozens, for sure. And in the back of my mind I feared that the same fate might be awaiting me.

Just as soon as I could I hurried over to Saira's place. If my father found out that I was helping Skip escape an arranged marriage, then I would be punished terribly. Once again, I would be rebelling against everything that he stood for. But I didn't care. I had to help Skip. Anyway, what worse was there he could do to me? Only kill me.

Saira was cut from the same cloth as Skip, and was also a rebel spirit. She had narrowly escaped a forced marriage herself. On learning of Skip's fate she was horrified. She agreed to help right away. Somehow, that very day she managed to get a flight ticket in Skip's name. She also managed to arrange for a friend who was visiting relatives to hand-carry it out to Pakistan.

Three days later I got a call from Saira. Skip had done it – she had escaped! She was safely back in the UK. She was at Saira's place right now, sleeping off her hideous ordeal. When I went to see Skip I realised how lucky she was to have escaped. Amazingly, her 'fiance' actually seemed sympathetic to her situation. He had given her back her passport, and driven her to the airport to help her get away. Without his help, she might never have made it.

Skip was shaken and shocked that her parents had tried to force her into such a marriage. She vowed never to speak to them again. She started working, rented her own flat, and cut herself off from them completely. But as far as Skip's parents were concerned, her actions had deeply 'dishonoured' the family, and so they didn't want any contact with her, either.

Skip's wasn't an isolated case. What made it so unusual was that she had managed to escape. All too often the trap of a forced marriage became a prison for life. Of course, everyone on the street knew what Skip had done. She was in absolute disgrace, they said. It was such a deep shame that she had brought on her family.

My father was especially vehement in his condemnation of Skip. He was gripped by a dark fury. How could a girl from his street, one of his 'flock', so defy her father's will? In my father's head the 'dishonour' was felt by the entire community, especially himself, the Imam, the community's moral and spiritual guide.

I didn't know if Skip's parents had spoken with Dad about setting up the forced marriage, but it's likely that they had. I kept quiet about my role in helping her escape. But at the same time I stayed in contact with her as best I could, although now it had to be a secret friendship. I admired her even more. Skip was my hero.

Skip loved poetry and writing and travel. She would work hard for a few months saving up her money, and then go off wherever she fancied. Every now and then she'd call me up from Egypt or Israel or some other place. She was always having such a great time. There was no real danger in her calling me at home. All she had to do was speak in English. Then my mum would just hand the phone to me.

'English-speaking girl,' she'd mutter, in Punjabi.

Skip's rebellion fuelled my own rebellious spirit, although my actions at twelve years old were a little less decisive. My hair was really long and it was all the same length. Every day I wore it in a big, thick plait. A couple of the girls on my street had their hair cut into fringes, and I thought it looked great. But Mum told me that it was bad and that Allah would punish them. Having a fringe was haram, she said.

I'd never read anything in the Quran that said it was wrong to cut your hair. The way Mum and Dad went on, everything was 'haram'. It was surprising that breathing was allowed! I thought fringes looked so fashionable, and I decided I was going to have one. I didn't care if it was 'haram'. I would just keep it secret. I always wore a hijab, even at home, so I'd just have to make sure my forbidden fringe was never visible.

One evening after school I went into the bathroom and locked the door. A lot of Muslims don't like to soak in the bath, because they think it's 'unclean'. You're lying in the water you've already made dirty. But it's not considered right to stand up to wash, either, so showering isn't on. Instead, we had a yellow plastic bucket that we filled up with water, and a plastic jug. We would crouch in the bath, and scoop up jug-fulls of water to pour over ourselves.

I got the yellow bucket so I could collect up my hair in it. I peered into the wooden framed mirror that sat over the sink. I took the pair of pink-handled scissors that I kept in my school pencil case, and took a lock of hair. Snip! The strand came away in my hand and I stared at it for a second. So easy. It was so easy to cut my hair. I dropped it into the bucket. It landed soundlessly. The thrill of rebellion! It felt so liberating.

Snip, snip, snip – on and on I went until finally I was done. I picked up the bucket, up-ended it over the loo, and flushed away the evidence. It was now that I started to feel worried and nervous. Once I emerged from the bathroom would Mum notice? I fiddled with my hijab, pulling it lower at the front. Then I opened the door and sneaked out of the bathroom.

I joined Mum in the kitchen. She didn't so much as glance at me. Why should she? With my forbidden fringe hidden by the scarf, I looked exactly the same as before. What a relief!

Some weeks later I was taking off my hijab before bed when Mum walked in. I tried to turn away but it was too late – she'd already caught sight of my DIY fringe.

'You stupid, stupid girl!' she cried. 'What have you done? Stupid girl. So worthless and stupid!'

She strode across to me and slapped me hard across the face.

'For doing that don't you know you'll be hung up by your hair in hell!' she cried. 'You'll burn in hell for it!'

I didn't say anything. I was shocked into silence by her actions. Mum had never hit me before. I knew that cutting my hair was supposed to be 'wrong', but not to that degree. When she cursed me to be hung up by my hair in hell, I feared that her curses might come true. Yet at the same time how could the simple act of cutting my hair be so sinful, I wondered. What harm had I done? How could it possibly have offended anyone's god?

I reckoned that I was going to hell anyway, if my parents' words were to be believed. A good Muslim is supposed to adhere to the Five Pillars of Islam if they are to reach Paradise, or so I had always been told. One of the Five Pillars is to pray five times a day, at the prescribed times. I was already failing in that by sneaking off to watch Neighbours instead. It looked as if mine was a lost cause, and that hell was where I was destined to end up.

Luckily, Mum didn't ever stay angry for long. And she didn't tell Dad about my evil, hair-cutting ways.

Poor Raz was still away in the Pakistani madrassa, and we had heard not a word from him. But Zakir and Billy were well into their teens by now, and they were also starting their own, small rebellions at home. One of our five daily prayers was supposed to be done at around the same time as the TV soap Neighbours, which was our favourite.

So, at around the time Neighbours came on my brothers and I would troop upstairs, as if we were off to pray. In fact, we would pile into Zakir's room and turn on the TV. As the oldest son, Zakir was allowed a TV in his room, although he'd had to save up the money from his Saturday job to buy it. If either brother tried complaining about having me in the room, I would threaten to tell Mum that they were actually watching a TV soap instead of praying. Together, we maintained a conspiracy of silence.

At first, I watched Neighbours simply because it was so much more interesting and fun. But by the time I was well into secondary school I had learned enough about other religions to start to question my own family's faith system. It was at this point that I first began to question whether I actually wanted to be a Muslim. But as far as I could see I was stuck in a religious ghetto, by birth and upbringing.

Dad seemed to get most of his sense of British culture from what we were watching on TV, which was more often than not the soaps. If people were shown drinking alcohol in a pub and flirting, he'd remark: 'Typical goray! That's all those English people ever do – drinking alcohol and sleeping around!'

As he had no direct experience of English culture, he chose to believe that the TV programmes were true to life. He believed that all *goray* behaved like that – regardless of what their faith was, or if they had no faith at all. If young people were shown talking back to their elders, he'd remark: 'Look! Look how they let their children do whatever they like! There's no respect in this society. No respect at all!'

Dad seemed to take great joy in anything that reinforced his prejudices, and that he could use to 'prove' his point. He paid special attention to the news whenever it was about youth crime, or young people binge-drinking. All of this served to reinforce what he believed about the people of his adopted country.

But what really got to him was if there were 'scantily clad' women on TV. If people were shown kissing, or even worse in bed together, he would blow a fuse. He'd shout at us to turn to another channel immediately. Even an instant's delay, and he would snap: 'Turn it over! Now!' No one would ever dream of refusing or challenging him. We knew how he would react if we did.

But it was still upsetting and frustrating. I used to think: *but I don't know what's going to happen now. They're just getting it together. That's a crucial part of the story. It's been building up to this for ages.*

Even if he let us turn back again – once the kissing and cuddling was over – we would still have missed a lot. I got used to trying to fill in the blanks with my imagination. Luckily, I was good at telling stories in my own head.

The more he disapproved, the more my brothers and I avidly watched the soaps. They were a window onto a different world: the typical northern community based around a pub, in Coronation Street; the tough guys in trouble with the police, in EastEnders; the students having free and easy love, in Hollyoaks. It was escapism. It was half an hour of thinking and feeling like other people – people free of the suffocating binds of our lives.

But in spite of Dad's fears, we didn't want to *be* like the characters in the soaps. I watched those soaps because I wanted to be a part of my friends' world. The soaps were a bridge between our separate realities. The soaps were the one thing that I could talk to my friends about that we shared. I couldn't talk to them about the other things that they did – holidaying, boyfriends, clothes, hairstyles or makeup. And I certainly couldn't share with them my dark and abusive home life. The soaps were our common ground.

Whenever Dad made us turn over during an important scene, I knew I would be missing a part my friends would have watched – and likely the juiciest bit. In school the next day they would all be talking about it, and I would be the one left out.

'You see EastEnders last night?' Lara would remark. 'Wow! Who'd have thought *they* were having an *affair*?'

Karen would laugh. 'Yeah, juicy, eh?'

'Who's having an affair?' I'd ask, eager to know the details I'd been forced to miss.

'You didn't watch it?' Karen would ask.

'I did, but not that bit.'

Karen would look confused. 'But why d'you always miss the best bits?'

'I'm not allowed to watch them!' I'd answer, angrily. 'My dad won't let me.'

'But why not?' Lara would ask. 'What's wrong with it?'

'It's all about religion,' I'd mutter, feeling utterly stupid to have to admit to such a thing. 'He says it's un-Islamic to see them.'

'But it's only kissing and stuff,' Karen would interject. 'They don't really *do* anything . . .'

Because my brothers and I went to an English school with English teachers and pupils, we understood English culture on a level that our parents could not. And yet at the same time we didn't quite feel part of it. We were 'in' England when we went to school, but we returned to the Pakistani village in the evenings. We had to learn to live a life split between two different worlds.

At school, I'd get told off for eating with my hand. At home, we never used cutlery. At home we spoke in Urdu or Punjabi, and Dad would get angry if I chatted with my brothers in English, the language of the despised goray. I even had a different vocabulary for my home life from that which I used at school.

In an attempt to build another bridge with my school friends I started getting into pop music in a big way. It was something else I could talk about at school. But inevitably this caused me trouble at home. The TV charts programme Top of the Pops was Dad's bête noir. He hated the music, the lyrics, the way people dressed, and the way they danced 'provocatively'. He ranted on and on about how it was such 'dirty dancing'.

But I used to ask myself, *how can it be so sinful?* How can it be fine for my father to abuse me in the cellar, when an innocent pop programme is so cursed? It made no sense to me. Dad's moral compass was so warped and awry. All I did know was that if Dad hated something, then I risked 'punishment' if I went against him. But I loved Top of the Pops, and still I watched it, especially if he was out.

I tried to learn the lyrics to the hit songs, so I could sing along with my friends. Mostly, they were about love – and it was the romantic kind of love between a man and a woman. To me romantic love seemed thrilling and mysterious. It was so wild and free compared to my parents' sterile and abusive coupling. I never once saw my father treat my mother with one iota of affection or appreciation. In reality, she was no better than a multi-function domestic appliance in his eyes.

When I looked at my parents there was nothing that spoke of love – not even the occasional soft word. Dad ordered Mum around and treated her like a slave, not as his equal and someone he was in love with. Instinctively, I knew this was wrong. I knew in my heart that he should be cherishing her. She was his wife, his life partner, and the mother of his children. But all she ever got from him was ignorance and violence.

I told myself that I didn't want to end up like Mum. But I could see older cousins and friends getting corralled into marriages that were equally loveless and stark. They didn't seem the remotest bit happy, or in love. In fact there was little that I could see that passed between men and women in our community that spoke of love.

Although I wasn't privy to what went on in every family home I never saw men and women showing any affection in public. No touching of any sort was allowed.

The sort of love in the pop song lyrics, the sort that I yearned for – that was part of the culture of my white friends. It wasn't part of my community, and in my parents' eyes it wasn't my destiny to find it, either.

With my teenage years all but upon me I felt trapped between two worlds. I didn't fit with my own culture, because I was drawn to that of my English friends. But I didn't fit into their culture, because I was a brown-skinned Muslim of Pakistani origin. I was far from happy with my Pakistani Muslim identity. In fact, I was starting to actively dislike it. But what was the alternative?

It didn't help that I was always dressed in a shalwar kamiz. Everyone wore it on my street, but whenever I was out of that environment I really hated having to wear it. Each month at school there were non-uniform days. Pupils were allowed to wear anything they wanted. Of course, the girls took this as an excuse to show off the newest fashions, and to doll themselves up in jewellery and makeup. But all I could ever wear was my canary yellow shalwar kamiz, with no makeup and jewellery. It made me feel even more like an outsider than I did the rest of the time.

Dad demanded that we dress 'modestly' at all times. This meant that even ankles weren't allowed to show. Exposed flesh, or tight clothes that suggested the shape of a woman's curves – these were sins of a great magnitude. I never tried to question this. If I did, Dad would see it as me being ashamed of our culture, and rebelling against his rule.

Dad said that for a woman to dress otherwise was unholy and ungodly. At the time, I didn't know that all this flesh- and hair-covering isn't compulsory under Islam. I had no great understanding of the rules of my faith, and in any case Dad was the Imam. Surely he had to know where the lines of what was allowed and what was forbidden were drawn.

Chapter Ten

Resistance, Sweet Resistance

Sunday afternoon was the time for the Radio One chart show, when I'd find out which song was Number One. Normally, I'd be in the bedroom ironing – so I could listen in with the volume turned right down. I had to keep an ear out for Dad, because if he caught me listening to the chart show I would be in trouble. I would snap off the radio at the slightest sound.

One of the rules of the house was that we weren't supposed to listen to music. According to Dad it was *haram* – forbidden. There was no explanation given as to why music was evil or ungodly. Ours was just a house officially bereft of music. Mum still listened to her Bollywood tapes, and Dad had his tapes of Pakistani qawwali singers. (Qawwali is similar to the chanting that whirling dervishes dance to, and is very popular in Pakistan.) Somehow their music wasn't haram, whereas our pop songs were.

Zakir and Billy were great fans of The Smiths and Morrissey. They'd listen late at night, or when Dad was at the mosque. They also loved watching Western movies, like Rebel Without A Cause. They got their fix of Western culture any way they could. Zakir always smelled of non-halal Fahrenheit aftershave. He loved his football, and was an avid fan of Manchester United. He never missed a match on TV.

Morrissey and The Smiths weren't the sort of music that I listened to. It was more grown-up and sophisticated rock music. But I still thought it was cool. Zakir and Billy had stickers on their wardrobes of Morrissey and James Dean looking full of attitude. One day the two of them decided to gel their hair into quiffs, just like their idols.

The first time they came downstairs with quiffs Dad looked at them strangely, but he didn't say anything. But they kept on doing it, and eventually Dad couldn't ignore it any longer. He didn't recognise or comprehend what they were doing, but he sensed the 'pollution' of his offspring with cursed Western ways. His sons' weird behaviour had to be confronted.

'What's that all about?' Dad snapped, jabbing a finger in the direction of Zakir's quiff. 'Long hair like a girl! It just looks stupid. So why do it?'

'It's nothing,' Zakir muttered. 'I just like it that way.'

'Well, it looks stupid,' Dad retorted. 'Gora hairstyles. What rubbish.'

In Dad's opinion the quiffs were a dangerous provocation. It was one step away from having long hair, which he hated. In his view males had to have closely shaven hair, in accordance with Islamic tradition. Huge bushy beards were a definite 'yes'; but long hair was a real 'no-no'. There was no way my brothers could tell him the truth – that they were trying to emulate their heroes, James Dean and Morrissey. That would have meant real trouble. Everyone was treading on eggshells in our household.

Morrissey was a vegetarian, and he had a song called 'Meat is Murder'. It was one of my brothers' favourites. Their next step in trying to be like him was to stop eating meat. One day they told Mum that they had become vegetarians. She started making them separate meals, or she just served them the vegetables. For a few weeks, Dad didn't seem to notice. But eventually – just as it was with the quiffs – Dad couldn't ignore what was going on.

'What's all this – not eating your meat?' he snorted. 'You'll never put on any weight or grow any muscles that way. How can you ever expect to be men?'

'What do you care?' retorted Billy, without thinking. 'We just don't want to eat it, that's all.'

Dad was furious, and there was a real argument. But he couldn't force his sons to eat, and there was no way he was ever going to understand that they wanted to be vegetarians. It was another source of mutual incomprehension between my father and his sons.

I thought their veggie act was really quite funny. I had a friend at secondary school who was a Hindu and a vegetarian by faith. Cows are sacred in Hinduism, and her family had decided not to eat meat of any kind. That made sense to me, but I just thought my brothers were being trendy. I'd heard them playing the Meat is Murder song, over and over. And I'd watched my brothers' video in which Morrissey had given a speech about not eating meat, and how chickens were kept in tiny cages.

Because Morrissey opposed battery farming, my brothers decided they wouldn't eat battery-farmed eggs, either. Mum would do anything for her sons, and so she started buying free-range eggs. The rest of us teased Billy and Zakir mercilessly. We'd sit at the dinner table and fish out juicy chunks of chicken from our curry. My little sister was the worst. She'd put the meat right under their nose.

'Mmm, doesn't that smell good?' she'd taunt them.

My mum's lamb sag – lamb and spinach curry – had always been Zakir's favourite. He especially liked it the second day after it had been cooked, in a toasted sandwich, when the spices had had time to marinate. So we started eating lamb sag toasted sandwiches right in front of Zakir, just to wind him up.

'It's so tender! And the spices – mmm, perfect!'

Of course, Dad failed to see the funny side of it. He ate in silence. Little did he know that his sons' vegetarianism was inspired by a rebellious white rock star. If he had realised it was this Western influence that lay behind it, he would have been even more angry. As it was he suffered his sons' 'aberrant' behaviour in a scowling, silent rage.

I couldn't openly rebel, like my brothers did. There was always the threat of 'punishment' to keep me cowed. I didn't try vegetarianism, and I always kept my tape cassettes of pop music well hidden. My sisters would try and grab my things and destroy them. Aliya used to get my schoolbooks and scribble all over them. The best hiding place was on top of the wardrobe, because she couldn't reach up there. It was also somewhere safe from Mum and Dad's prying.

By now there were four of us sleeping in the one bedroom – Mum, Sabina, Aliya and me. We each had one shelf in the wardrobe for our clothes. There were no posters or pictures on the walls, just more of the 1970s-style flowery wallpaper that we had in the lounge. One night I had a whole conversation with Sabina when she was fast asleep. Like Mum, Sabina adored Bollywood music, but she always kept her tapes hidden. Knowing Sabina was talking in her sleep I decided to play a trick on her.

'Where did you put your music tapes?' I asked her.

'In a box under the bed,' she replied, in a voice that sounded a bit weird.

The next morning I told her just where her precious Bollywood tapes were. I told her she'd been talking in her sleep and that's how I'd found them. Sabina was so annoyed. For once I had an advantage over my parents' perfect little daughter! She rushed upstairs to check, and I relished the fact that I had tricked her. After that she had to change her hiding place, for she knew I had discovered it.

Even the smallest rebellion had to be hidden, and not just from my parents. If Sabina found something out, she'd right away tell on me. We were like chalk and cheese, and we just didn't get along. She was my dad's perfect daughter, whilst I was the rebellious, cursed one – the one who deserved only his abuse and rage.

I had a school pencil case on which I had written my friends' names in Tipp-Ex. Hidden inside were stickers of pop stars and actors from the Smash Hits magazine. My favourites were Bros, New Kids on the Block, and the stars of the TV series Beverly Hills 90210. I had a crush on Luke Perry, one of the actors in that show. He was tall, slim and handsome, with blue eyes and sandy hair. I thought he was gorgeous.

My parents never went through my school stuff, so my stickers were safe in there. In fact they rarely if ever showed any interest in my schooling. But one time my little sister got hold of my school bag and caused havoc. She ripped out all the stickers, and wrote all over my posters. Eventually, Mum caught her scribbling on a wall. Aliya was too young to realise that the contents of my school bag were haram – forbidden. But I was still really upset. My school bag was the entirety of my private life, and I had to defend it against everyone.

Another time Zakir and Billy got hold of my pencil case. They thought it was hilarious. Bros were a cheesy pop band for little girls, and they thought I was really sad for liking them. They laughed at me for trying to hide the stickers, and told me to stop being such a girl. And they teased me about my crush on Luke Perry for weeks on end.

I was so angry with them. 'What are you looking at? It's secret! Who said you could go in my bag!'

The more annoyed I got, the more that egged them on to jeer and laugh at me. But at least I knew they wouldn't tell Dad. We all had our secrets, and in a way we protected each other. I knew things they were getting up to that Dad didn't. They would go to pop concerts, whilst telling Dad that they were going out to visit one of the neighbours on our street. They even had copies of the New Musical Express in their bedroom. So if they told on me, they knew I could cause them trouble, too.

When my oldest brother, Zakir, turned eighteen he started working full-time and got himself a car. It was a second-hand purple Skoda, but still it was his pride and joy. He was forever getting me or my sisters to wash and polish it. If we refused, he'd say he wasn't taking us anywhere in it. He only ever took us to the shops to get the groceries, but at least that saved us having to carry the heavy bags home.

The Skoda was at least an improvement on Mum's wheelie shopping cart. My parents had never owned a car. What did they need one for, when all they ever did was stay in the house, walk around our street or to the mosque, or undertake their yearly visit to Pakistan? They had never learned to drive. In Pakistan they had used a horse and cart. And in the UK Dad used to walk everywhere.

One winter it snowed heavily, and Dad came home having hurt his knee. He wouldn't tell anyone how he had injured it, because he was too embarrassed to admit that he had slipped in the snow. He kept walking on it, until it was too painful. Only then did he relent and let Mum and Zakir take him to hospital. After an X-ray and various other tests the doctors concluded that it was badly sprained. It was swathed in bandages, after which Dad used to get Zakir to drive him to the mosque. Nothing was allowed to get in the way of his duties as the Imam.

Of course, a Skoda wasn't the glitziest of cars by any means, but to Zakir it was a real status symbol. It wasn't so impressive to me. My friends at school had older brothers with Peugeots or Volkswagens – and I quickly realised that just about anything was better than a Skoda.

'You can drive me anywhere,' I used to tell Zakir, 'just don't pick me up from school!'

Zakir seemed to find this very funny. One day I came out of school to hear the loud beeping of a car horn. And there was Zakir, waving out of the window of the purple Skoda, a big cheesy grin on his face. My friends fell about laughing. I pretended not to know him. But my sister Sabina immediately saw a way of getting back at me. She had just started at the secondary school. She grabbed my arm and dragged me over to the car. There was no way I could disown Zakir and his purple Skoda now.

Earlier that year the school had taken us on a coach trip to see the switching-on of the Blackpool lights. This was the furthest that I had ever been from home, apart from the one visit to Pakistan. From year to year we never left my home town. It was also the first time that I'd ever seen the sea. We drove along the sea front and through the town, gawping at the fancy illuminations. As for the sea, there was a fleeting glimpse of rippling light on darkened waters, and that was it.

That Easter holiday I asked Zakir if he would drive me and my sisters to Blackpool, so we could see the sea properly. For some reason I used to daydream about the sea – this vast expanse of water I could barely imagine existing for real. It had captured my imagination, as if somehow its watery vastness might offer calm in my troubled world.

But Zakir refused take us. He acted as if he just didn't want to go, but I reckoned he was afraid of what Dad might say. For all we knew Dad might have deemed such a venture haram. Who knew what supposed religious edicts he might cook up to prevent us from fulfilling our dreams.

The fact that Zakir refused to take us meant there was to be no relief from the boredom and trauma of home that Easter. I tried to spend as much time as possible out of the house. One afternoon I was coming home from my Uncle Kramat and Auntie Sakina's place. I was late getting home to pray, and I came rushing up our street. As I went to turn into the front yard I slipped and collided with the gatepost, collapsing onto the ground in a heap.

After a few seconds I got to my feet, and found there was blood streaming down my face from a gash on my forehead. Auntie Sakina's daughter was gossiping with Mum on the doorstep. As soon as they saw the state of me they knew I needed to get to hospital. Auntie Sakina's son, Uncle Ahmed, rushed me there in his car. After a short wait in Casualty I was stitched up and allowed to go home. Mum didn't say very much more about it. I went to bed, feeling exhausted from the shock and the loss of blood.

When I came downstairs the next morning Dad's expression said it all for me. He didn't show the slightest hint of concern, or sympathy. Instead, he looked at me as if I was the most stupid thing on earth. His disdain – no, his *disgust* – for his daughter wasn't going to be alleviated by a bad knock to the head.

It was just one more occasion when Dad told me how stupid and useless I was.

Chapter Eleven

Rebel with a Cause

I don't know whether it was Skip's example or not, but at the age of thirteen I really began to question why my world was like it was. How could my life be so abusive, and so dark? Why was my spirit so crushed with drudgery? I started to question everything around me: my culture, my family, my father, my religion, and of course the abuse.

As I grew, my father's perverse desires seemed more inflamed by my pubescent body. It was only by being at school, or being at out of the house as much as possible, that I managed to avoid him for any significant amount of time. But always there came a moment when he'd catch me at home with the right excuse to visit his 'punishment' on me.

He'd force me to take off my clothes, watching me in the dim cellar lamplight as I did so. By the time I had removed every last item, he'd be panting heavily, his breath coming in gasps. His eyes would be full of that terrifying, crazed animal lust that I'd seen so often before. He'd hitch up his robe and force me to touch him. I had no choice but do so, for if I tried to refuse he'd punch and kick me to the floor. And when I did touch him he'd start muttering away in Punjabi about me being a 'worthless, dirty girl' and a 'dirty, evil temptress and a whore'.

Later, after he'd tired of raping me, he'd order my mother to let me out, by unlocking the door. He couldn't even bear to see me after he'd 'punished' me. He just didn't want to have me around, for I was a living reminder of his evil ways. I'm sure he would have been happier then if I was dead, for alive I was a rebuke to him. Whenever he was forced to come face to face with me he'd turn on me, in front of whoever was there – my mum, my sisters, whoever – and slap me.

'You'll never find a husband,' he'd snarl at me, 'because you're too ugly, and stupid! Who'd ever want you? You're not good enough for anyone!'

I'd stare at the floor in silence.

'See,' he'd hiss at Sabina. 'I'm teaching her a lesson for being dirty and stupid. But I'm sure you'll never follow in her evil ways.'

My dysfunctional family didn't make the slightest sense to me. The natural love of a child for her parents, and her parents' love for her, was non-existent. In fact, in my case it seemed never to have existed. I couldn't for one moment understand how Mum could be complicit in Dad's evil behaviour. Why did she allow it? It was beyond me.

As for Dad, I was starting to realise just how much I hated and loathed him. No longer was I living in the hope that he might somehow change. I no longer lived for the day when he would 'forgive' me and accept me and love me as his daughter. I knew that would never happen. And rather than me being the 'evil' one, I knew that the real darkness lay all in him.

The older I got the less I seemed to believe in the same things as my family. But at the same time, I didn't know what else to believe in. I was not like the rest of them. I spent a lot of time on my own, writing in my diary. I found myself communicating with my family less and less. At 5.30 in the afternoon, one or other of the boys would go with Dad to the mosque, to issue the call to prayer. But I would head upstairs to watch Neighbours. Sometimes Mum would check on me to see if I was praying, but by now I had learned well how to lie.

'Yes, Mum,' I'd sigh in answer to her inevitable question. 'I've just done my prayers.' Really, I'd been watching Scott marry Charlene.

At school we were now learning about other world religions. Until this point, I had learned little in any detail about Judaism, Buddhism or Hinduism. Now I had the chance to consider properly how there were many different paths of religious thought, and many different world belief systems. Our RE teacher was a white lady in her fifties. She talked about each religion with the same degree of respect, as if she favoured neither one nor the other. She gave the impression that the major faiths of the world were a menu from which those amongst us so-inclined could choose.

A lot of my school friends had no faith – or at least, if they did, it didn't manifest itself in any noticeable way at school. Some of them didn't even believe in the existence of God. I wasn't particularly shocked by this. It was just how they thought, and that was fine by me. Whatever their faith or lack of it they were lovely to me, and they were my friends.

Dad found atheism, and all other religions other than Islam, abhorrent. As he saw it, Islam was the one true faith. But I was intrigued by different belief systems and ideas. I loved hearing people talk about them. I had been reared by xenophobic and intolerant parents, living in a closed community – and yet that hadn't poisoned my own view of the world. There was something in my nature that opened my mind, and made me curious and searching.

In our RE lessons we were taught about people converting from one religion to another. To me, this was a revolutionary idea. Until then, I had just assumed that you were born into a religion, and that would remain your belief system until you died. It was inconceivable in my community to convert out of Islam. Once I heard a story on the street about someone who had done so. It was told to us as a dark warning. People were up in arms about it. The only thing good enough for converts, they said, was death. Those who turned their backs on the one true faith deserved only to die.

One thing that I really started to question was why I had to pray in Arabic. In the school library I had seen an English translation of the Quran, but I knew Dad wouldn't allow me to read it. Dad insisted that the Quran as rendered in Arabic was the exact recording of Allah's word. Translation corrupted the word of God, and the Quran didn't have any 'spiritual truth' in other languages. The fact that none of us – Dad, the Imam, included – understood Arabic didn't seem to concern him.

The result of this was that I – like everyone else on my street – had little idea what the scriptures actually said. All I knew was the teachings that Dad and a handful of other religious leaders allowed me to hear. I had access to a school Bible in English, and, sensing my interest, my RE teacher began showing me other religious texts that I could read: the Eight-fold Path of Buddhism; the Bhagavad-Gita of Hinduism; and the Torah of Judaism.

After all my years of Quran study, I was finally reading religious texts that actually made sense to me. *They spoke to me.* Some of the teachings did, too. I loved the story of the Good Samaritan. The contrast with my own faith, where I didn't understand a thing, could not have been more pronounced.

I found myself interested in what these other religions had to say, and about the relationship those who believed had with their God. Whilst in my upbringing Islam had always been about submission – and in our case, dumb submission – many of these other faiths seemed to be truly enlightening. Adherents sought a personal, uplifting relationship with their God, one based wholly upon understanding his or her holy message.

I was full of confusion. Why did we Muslims pray five times a day in Arabic, when we didn't understand a word of those prayers? Why did we mumble words in incomprehension? I'd heard other Muslims say that when they prayed in Arabic they felt an inner peace. But I didn't feel any such thing. I never gave voice to my misgivings over my faith, but my RE teacher could sense it, and she could tell that I was interested in all faiths. She appreciated that, and fed my hunger to learn.

I never once brought this interest home with me. Dad had said that we weren't even allowed to mention Jesus' name at home. Likewise, I expected that these other faith systems would be blindly condemned by my father

One day when I was walking home from school I heard a terrible commotion outside Jack the Jack Russell's house. It sounded like someone was screaming. I turned to look, and there was a white man in Jack's owner's garden, brandishing a knife. I didn't recognise him, but he was shouting wildly, and he looked somehow unhinged.

I ran towards my house in a panic. As soon as I was inside I grabbed the phone, and without thinking I rang the police. They asked for the address where the trouble was, and then they started asking for my details. I panicked, and put the phone down.

No one in our community had much contact with the police. There was a Pakistani Muslim police officer living on a neighbouring street, and people would always go to him in the first instance if there was any trouble, for he was one of our own. The community as a whole trusted and respected him.

Like most people on the street, my parents feared 'outsiders' coming in and upsetting their ways. The police were seen as outsiders, not as people who would protect you if things went wrong. In Pakistan, the police are renowned for being corrupt, and generally dealings with them are best avoided. Most people on my street presumed the British police were pretty much the same.

Shortly after my making that emergency call, a police car rolled up in front of our house. A couple of uniformed officers knocked on the door. Mum answered, and they told her what had happened, with me acting as translator. They had traced the phone call. I could see the look of shock on her face. The police must have thought she was scared, but I knew better. She just knew it was me who had made the call, and she was angry.

There was no point in not owning up to it, so I told the police exactly what had happened. They didn't seem to mind. They just told me that if there was a next time then I should stay on the line and give my name and address. It was important that they got any potential witness's details. They went across the road to investigate. I wasn't scared of the police any more – I was scared of how my parents were going to react.

As soon as the police were gone, Mum unleashed her anger on

me. But it was nothing compared to what happened when she told my father. Why had I rung the 'goray police', Dad demanded. Why was I interfering? Why was I getting into other people's business? Jack's owner was a gori, she wasn't one of us. I should have left it well alone.

Jack's owner might live on our street, but she was white and English and that's what mattered. It made her an outsider. If someone attacked her with a knife, that was their business. It wasn't a danger to us or ours. Let her deal with it. I knew that I had done the right thing, but my parents warned me never to phone the police again.

As they ranted on at me, they expected their blind prejudice and unreasoning fear to seep into my mind. The police were dangerous outsiders, they said. They were corrupt, and looked after their own. Fear and prejudice piled on fear and prejudice, until I wished for all the world that I had never rung the police in the first place. I was sure I would never call them again.

Afterwards, I couldn't help dwelling on what had happened. On one hand, I knew what I had done was morally right. It could have saved Jack's owner's life. But on the other, here were my parents telling me that the police were against us, and that people's lives weren't our concern unless they were Pakistani Muslims.

Again, I was confused. I was starting to question the mores of my community – where someone might be left to be knifed just because they weren't 'one of us'. What sort of people behaved like that? In my mind my community and my religion were inextricably linked. Jack's owner wasn't just a gori. She wasn't just English. She was also a non-Muslim.

For the first time I began seriously to consider running away. I had had enough of Dad's abuse, and enough of being treated as the family slave in a dysfunctional home. And I was starting to lose my faith in my community and my religion. But where could I run? There was nowhere that I could find sanctuary. Outside of my family and my street, I didn't have one single relative or friend who could offer me sanctuary.

I knew that if I did try to run away and was caught, the

consequences would be unthinkable. I knew what happened to girls in our community who tested the boundaries by making a desperate bid for freedom. They were immediately sent 'back' to Pakistan, and forced into marriage. And from there they never returned.

And so it was that I began to consider the most drastic option possible – that of ending it all. Every Saturday we watched the TV drama Casualty, and that was what first gave me the idea of committing suicide, and how I might go about doing it.

Although Dad hadn't been beating Mum for years now, she still suffered from chronic headaches. He had stopped hitting her when he started to beat and abuse me. I had taken the heat of his evil and anger, but Mum still suffered from stress-related migraines. She still felt trapped, and fearful of Dad's rage. And she would get horribly upset whenever she knew he was abusing me. She would try to hide it, but in her heart she knew full well what was going on down in the cellar, and it tore her apart.

Whenever Dad indulged his sick desires with me, Mum would develop these terrible headaches. To relieve the pain, she took heaps of paracetamol. There were lots of packets in a drawer in the kitchen. We were also allowed to take them if we felt ill.

I rescued a little plastic pillbox from the rubbish bin, and started to store painkillers in it. I removed the paracetamol very, very carefully, sneaking them away one by one. That way I felt certain Mum wouldn't know. In any case, with eight of us in the house I knew that no one could ever pin it on me. Gradually, I built up a stock of the small white tablets. I hid the box amongst my clothes on my shelf in the wardrobe.

I hadn't resolved to kill myself yet, but I was getting more and more desperate. I couldn't see any other way out. My stock of paracetamol was the last resort. If I reached a point where I couldn't go on, I knew they were there and that I could take them. They were the promise of my final release from the predations of my father.

I was approaching fourteen years old by now. Had I been told at this point that I was being packed off to a marriage in Pakistan, there is no doubt in my mind that I would have taken every last one of those pills. They were my insurance policy. It was dark and desperate relief, but a relief all the same just knowing they were there.

As I got older, non-uniform days became a bigger and bigger deal. There was a fashion for 'shell suits' – garishly coloured shiny nylon tracksuits. Girls used to wear them with huge hoop earrings, and their hair done up in ponytails. As for the makeup, they really used to cake it on. I dreaded the non-uniform days. All I ever had to wear was my dull shalwar kamiz and headscarf, in bright canary yellow. I felt mortified going to school in this outfit, when everyone else dressed as they liked. I thought I looked exactly like I was – like a caged bird.

My friends knew I hated it, so they pretended not to notice. But those who didn't know me weren't so kind. Sometimes I got called horrible names by pupils from other classes. I was already a shy girl, and having people yell 'Paki!' at me in the corridors didn't help very much. All I wanted to do was fit in.

I wished and wished for all the world that I had a shell suit. I dreamt of wearing a shiny turquoise one, with bright pink lipstick and blue eyeshadow. I just knew I would look great dressed like that.

With Skip having moved away from our street I befriended Sonia, a petite and very pretty girl with long black hair and wide brown eyes. Sonia was in the same class as my sister, Sabina, so she was three years younger than me. But otherwise, she wasn't the least bit like my conformist sister. Like Skip, Sonia had a rebel spirit, and that's what drew us together.

Sonia's house was a terraced Victorian one a little like ours. It was located halfway between our street and the school bus stop. Her parents were from India, and they had been living in Britain for about as long as mine. But unlike my parents, they both spoke excellent English. And they worked out and about in the wider community – her father as an office worker, her mother as a nurse. They had chosen to be a part of the culture of the country they called home, in contrast to my mum and dad.

Both Sonia and I had been called 'Pakis' by racist people, at one time or another. Yet there were huge differences between Sonia's family of professional, middle-class Indians, and my family of unskilled rural dwellers. Sonia's folks came from a big city, as opposed to a dusty backwater, so they were used to the urban lifestyle. And Sonia's family's attitude towards women was completely different from that of my own. Sonia's grandmother had been a medical doctor in India, and it was normal and expected for women to get educated, to work and be independent.

Sonia's life was much freer than my own. She was allowed to go down town, to meet her friends and hang out. She was always dressed in Western clothes. No one made her wear a sari or a shalwar kamiz. As an only child she was under pressure from her parents to get good grades. But at least they backed her one hundred per cent in her schooling, as opposed to my own. Her mum was always going on about how Sonia's nose was too big, and there was even talk of her having plastic surgery.

Once we'd got to know each other well, Sonia talked to me about her 'problems'. She had almost started to believe that her nose was too big, and she worried that it made her ugly. She would get stressed out at exam times, in case she let her parents down. I tried to be sympathetic, but it was clear to me she had absolutely nothing to worry about. I talked to her in turn about some of my problems. I told her how I hated wearing shalwar kamiz, and how I was banned from meeting my friends down town.

But I kept the real darkness hidden. I couldn't bring myself to talk about the way Dad had been beating and abusing me for the last eight years. It was too dark and too dirty, and at some level I felt guilty and ashamed of what was happening. There was no way I could bring myself to open up about that shame with anyone. I would have felt far too vulnerable and exposed. And I feared I would lose a lovely friend – if she discovered how dirty and sick was my secret home life.

So I complained instead about having nothing to wear on non-uniform day.

'Well, there's an easy way around that,' Sonia declared, with a mischievous grin. 'Tomorrow's a non-uniform day, isn't it? Come to my house on the way to school. My parents leave early for work. You and I are about the same size, so you can wear my clothes. We can dress up together!'

Wow! I was thrilled. I didn't even consider the risk. I just thought of being able to go to school for once in my life not wearing shalwar kamiz. The next morning I left the house fifteen minutes early. I hurried over to Sonia's place and knocked on the door.

'Ready? Come on!' Sonia declared, as she opened the door and pulled me in.

Her house was simply lovely. We passed through a modern-looking kitchen in golden yellow pine, which was dominated by a big dining table and chairs. Then there was a living room in plain pastel shades. I noticed a picture on the wall of the Taj Mahal, an incredibly beautiful building in India, whose white towers and facades are reflected in a mirror-like pool. I recognised it from my RE lessons, in which we were taught that it is a place with both Hindu and Islamic origins.

Upstairs, Sonia had her own room. It was neat and tidy compared to the crowded bedroom at home. Sonia had posters on the walls that I immediately recognised – they were of actors from Beverly Hills 90210, my favourite TV series. The series depicts the lives of a group of rich high school kids in America. It tells the stories of their friendships, romances and dramas. All of my school friends watched it, and we'd gossip over the twists and turns of the plot, and what boys we liked.

I told Sonia that I wanted to marry Luke Perry – the star of the show. I kept his picture in my pencil case. She told me that she had a crush on one of his co-stars, Jason Priestley. So that was all right – we weren't going to end up fighting over the same man! There would have been no point anyway: Sonia was far more beautiful than I could ever hope to be.

We rifled through Sonia's clothes as quickly as we could. She had simple tastes, but her clothes were Western and fashionable

– so to me they were lovely, and as exotic as could be. I chose a pair of tight jeans and a plain T-shirt. As I pulled on those jeans I felt a delicious frisson of excitement. This was the first time in my life that I'd ever worn a pair of trousers, and felt denim next to my skin. It was also the first time in many years that I would be going outside minus my Islamic head-covering.

I stuffed my shalwar kamiz and hijab into my school bag. Before leaving there was just time to do our makeup – eyeliner, mascara, and a smear of red lipstick. Mum had made me up once or twice before, when we went to weddings at the mosque, so I had some idea of what to do. Sonia showed me the rest. Then she did my hair. We looked in the mirror above her dressing table, and decided that we looked great!

On the way out Sonia showed me the spare bedroom. In one corner there was a little shrine: a statue of a man with the head of an elephant, surrounded by candles and incense.

'That's a Hindu god, isn't it?' I said. I recognised it from RE lessons, but couldn't remember the name.

'It is. It's Ganesh,' said Sonia. 'This is where my parents pray. They put offerings of food and money into that little dish.'

I noticed that Sonia had said it was where her *parents prayed*. She made it sound as if she didn't have to. I didn't pry, but I guessed her parents' religion was a lot less strict than my own.

As we went to step out of her house, I felt a momentary shudder of terror. Could I really do this, I wondered. I held back, hovering on the doorstep.

'Sonia, what if someone sees me?' I hissed.

She smiled at me. 'Come on! You look great. And no one will notice . . . Anyway, we've got to go now or we'll be late for school!'

I was certain that someone from the community would spot me. I felt so conspicuous. But as we stepped out of the house and made our way to the bus stop no one seemed to pay us any attention. We reached the bus stop, and suddenly there were Amina and Ruhama, two of the girls from my street. When they saw me, they did a double take.

'Wow! Hannan, is that you?' Amina asked.

'Where did you get those clothes?' Ruhama added.

'None of your business,' I replied sharply, with a hint of a threat in my voice.

I didn't want anyone making a fuss for two reasons. Firstly, I didn't want it getting out that I had gone to school dressed like a gora. Amina and Ruhama were allowed to dress like that, but I wasn't and everyone knew it. The less fuss they made, the better. Secondly, I was so embarrassed that I had had to borrow someone else's clothes. I really wanted to keep that quiet. Otherwise, everyone on the bus would hear, and it would soon get around school.

Part of me worried that Amina and Ruhama would go home and tell their parents that they had seen me, the Imam's daughter, dressed like a real gori! The fact that I had gone to school wearing makeup and no hijab would be great gossip on our street – some of the best, in fact. What a juicy scandal! Before I had even got to school I was worried about the news getting back to my father. But I wasn't about to stop now. I was determined to feel normal for just one day, whatever might happen afterwards.

We reached the school gates, and for the first time in my life I wasn't embarrassed at what I was wearing. I had *chosen* to dress like this. It was such a joyful, liberating feeling.

My friends didn't make a big deal of it. They had accepted me in my shalwar kamiz, and now they just seemed to accept the changed me as well. All they said was: 'Wow, you look good!' And if any of the teachers were aware of my changed appearance, none of them said so. Of course, there was one person who made nasty comments – my younger sister, Sabina.

'Why are you dressed like that?' she demanded. Her face was twisted into a sneer. 'Where did you get that stuff – that *gori stuff*?'

Sabina was speaking in Punjabi, so that none of the others could understand her.

'It's Sonia's,' I replied, deliberately speaking in English. 'Got a problem?'

'She's a *Hindu*,' said Sabina, turning up her nose. 'Why are you wearing a Hindu's stuff?'

*

'What does it matter?' I retorted. 'I like these clothes, and I'm going to carry on wearing them.'

I was gambling that Sabina wouldn't risk spilling the beans on me at home. If she did, I would tell all her friends that she was a snitch. At home, Sabina was a snitch by nature, but no one liked snitches at school. That's why I had replied to her in English. It was a thinly veiled threat. It was a way of saying – *you tell on me at home, and I'll tell on you at school.*

All that day I felt just great. At last I really felt like one of the girls. Sonia and I had worked out a plan of action for after school, in case Zakir or Mum was waiting for me. Sonia went first and checked. If Zakir was there, she was to come back in and alert me, and I would change into my shalwar kamiz in the girls' toilets. If Mum was there, we reckoned we could sneak past without her noticing.

Sonia told me the coast was clear. We got the bus home and walked back to her house, where I did my transformation in reverse. Off came the jeans and the T-shirt, off came the makeup. The hair went back into a plait. I put the canary yellow shalwar suit back on, and replaced the hijab on my head. I arrived back on my street dressed exactly as I had left it. No one gave any sign that they knew about my subterfuge.

This was the most delicious rebellion that I'd yet experienced, and it both thrilled and frightened me. From now on, whenever it was non-uniform day I did the dressing-up routine at Sonia's house. Sonia had become my partner in crime. She didn't have any sisters, and she enjoyed us dressing up together. She was also aware that she was doing something 'forbidden' – or, at least, something that was forbidden to me. She didn't seem worried about what would happen if we got found out. She knew that I would be the one to get into trouble, not her.

I didn't want to think about what my parents would do if they found out. Dad's anger would know no bounds. I'd face a savage beating, and worse. But I was willing to take that risk. The reward was a simple, blissful sense of freedom, and that was incredibly valuable to me. Everything else in my life seemed to be beyond my control: who I worshipped, how I worshipped, what I thought, how I was treated physically as the *de facto* family slave. Even my own body was someone else's to control and misuse in horrible ways.

At last, I had managed to do something that was by my choice, and under my control.

I wasn't about to give that up very easily.

Chapter Twelve

The Outsider

Shortly after my fourteenth birthday my brother Raz walked back into our lives. Raz had been gone for over three years, and there had been no warning that he was coming home. Mum hugged him welcome, and straight away Raz burst into tears. He carried on sobbing for what seemed like an age, as Mum tried to comfort and quiet him. I was shocked by Raz's appearance, and how troubled he seemed.

Raz was like a completely different person after his time in that Pakistani madrassa. He looked old beyond his years and painfully thin. But worst of all he seemed to have lost all of his confidence and joy in life. The sparkle and laughter had gone out of his eyes. It was like a light had been turned off, the brightness being replaced by a vacant, empty darkness. Poor Raz. What had they done to him, I wondered.

Over the days that followed I tried to laugh with Raz about the things he'd always found funny – like Mum doing her Cockney accent during EastEnders, or Zakir and Billy's vegetarianism. But even that didn't raise a smile. He didn't speak a word to me about what had happened over the previous three years. He just refused to talk about it.

But one day we heard about a friend of Raz's who was scheduled to go to a Pakistani madrassa shortly.

'He mustn't go!' Raz blurted out. 'Don't let him go. He'll hate it there. It'll kill him . . .'

Mum didn't know what to say.

'Why? Why will he hate it?' I ventured. 'What's so bad about it, Raz?'

Raz looked at the floor. 'It's bad because they beat you up,' he murmured. 'It's bad because they beat you if you get it wrong. And they don't just hit you with a stick, like in the mosque. They smash you to the floor, and you are punched and kicked for hours on end. It's torture. That's what they do. They torture you . . .'

I listened in growing horror as Raz continued. 'One day, I failed to get the pronunciation of one of the Surahs right. I kept trying, but I just couldn't do it perfectly. So they beat me up and then they locked me in a horrible, dark room for days on end. *You'll stay in there until you learn to do it properly,* they said, *and you'll die in there if you don't.* And there were other things too . . .'

Raz's voice trailed off into nothing. He was haunted by the memories. I could see the fear in his eyes. He didn't want to say more.

'I never, ever want to go back there,' Raz said, at last. 'If anyone tries to send me back I'll kill myself first . . .'

The old, fun-loving Raz was gone. That Raz had been broken down and torn apart in that place that my father had sent him to. Instead, he had been remade as a closed and wounded young man whose love of life had been destroyed. Well done, Dad, I told myself. He had managed to remake Raz in something like his own image. In adult life Raz would develop serious psychological problems. I don't know whether his time in the madrassa triggered it, but I do know that it left him with horrible scars.

What happened to Raz is the same as happens in many madrassas in Pakistan, in which they prepare boys to fight a 'jihad' against the West. They take them from their families at a vulnerable age, and torture them and break their spirit. Then, when the boys can be controlled, they indoctrinate them with hatred and send them off as cannon fodder to fight. At least Raz had escaped that fate. But he had been pushed a long way down that lonely, dark and brutalising road.

Where my happy-go-lucky brother had once been there was now little more than a shadow. Whilst talking to Raz it occurred to me that my father had gone to a similar madrassa when he was a boy. Perhaps that might explain some of his warped, perverted, violent ways. But it didn't excuse them. Nothing could ever do that.

Shortly after Raz's return trouble flared up in the Middle East. Iraq had invaded Kuwait, and the Gulf region descended into war. This was a difficult time for us. At the top of our street the council had built a smart new college for those with learning disabilities and the long-term unemployed.

There was resentment on our street that 'they' – the disabled and the 'dolies' – were coming into our street. The community avoided having any contact with them. Most of the adults saw them as being the 'dregs' of English society.

In the mindset of many in my parents' generation a child with a disability was seen as being a curse from Allah. It was a sign that Allah was punishing you for some sin you had committed. It was a 'shame' on the entire family. In the rural areas of Pakistan children born with disabilities were often 'got rid of'. Or, if they lived, they would be hidden away inside the house, sometimes for their entire lives.

This attitude informed how people on my street viewed people with disabilities. There was little sense that we might have sympathy for them, or try to see them as fellow human beings.

Skip's oldest sister, Zaria, had a disabled daughter. Her limbs were weak, and she was unable to support herself. I had seen how the rest of the community treated that child. If there was a gathering at their house, Zaria's family would hide the little girl away in one of the bedrooms. It was as if she didn't exist. Zaria's family loved that little girl, but they just couldn't break out of the constraints of religion and tradition.

Sometimes, on the rare occasions that I managed to get around to Skip's house, her disabled niece might be there. If she was, Skip and I would play with her. Contact with her was how I learned that my community's view of people with disabilities was wrong. From then on whenever I saw children in wheelchairs I wouldn't think that they were 'untouchables', or shameful in any way.

There was always tension on college days, when the disabled and the dolies would arrive on 'our' street. And there was always a palpable sense of relief when their day was over and they were gone. The people with disabilities were 'shameful', and the dolies were low-life. This was the height of hypocrisy, of course. Plenty of people on our street – my father included – were on benefits. But there was supposedly a difference between them and us.

In my father's case he was the Imam, which rendered him immune from 'dolie' status. At first it had been easy for Dad to claim the dole. But recently the authorities had started insisting that all claimants do training programmes or classes. You had to be an active job-seeker, not just a passive 'dolie'. However, if you were on a 'sickie', that was like being on one extended holiday.

As they tightened up the rules, Dad decided to 'do a sickie'. He used the excuse that he had hurt his back. It was true that he did have a bad back, but that didn't mean he couldn't work. It certainly didn't stop him from officiating at the mosque on a daily basis. He could have learned to speak English, and that might have made him more employable. He could have learned to drive, and become a taxi driver. But as far as Dad was concerned nothing was going to stop him from claiming benefits for himself and the entire family, while continuing to work as the community Imam.

Dad didn't see himself as a 'slacker'. He didn't seem to feel the slightest bit of guilt that his entire eight-person family survived on benefits. Far from it. Somehow, he saw no moral dilemma in taking money from a state that he despised, in order to be the spiritual guide of his community. It was all perfectly justifiable in his mind.

But the dolies from the college were something different. They wore ripped jeans and leather jackets, and the men sported earrings. A number of them had 'skinhead' haircuts. In between classes they stood outside the college, smoking or drinking alcohol – cheap canned lager, or cider in plastic bottles.

My 'quiffed' brothers Billy and Zakir might have secretly thought the dolies looked cool. But the fact they didn't have jobs wasn't cool at all. Despite the family's reliance on benefits, my brothers had a strong work ethic. Whilst the older generation felt that their lives had advanced hugely from where they had started out, the younger generation wanted to 'advance' a lot more! The idea that being a dropout was cool was anathema. Everyone wanted to get ahead, and the dolies represented everything that was abhorred.

Most of the time the dolies just ignored us. But I would feel scared walking past them, especially if they'd been drinking. Then they'd be laughing and swearing loudly, and it was innately threatening behaviour. But they didn't call us names or abuse us physically. Or at least, not yet.

When the fighting began in the Gulf War, all that began to change.

Whenever we walked past they would yell out: 'Paki! Saddam-lover! Bloody Paki!'

The fact that our families hailed from Pakistan, a part of Asia, and that we weren't Iraqi Arabs, seemed lost on them. We were brown-skinned and Muslim, and that was enough. One day I was walking past with my eldest brother, Zakir, when a group of skinheads turned their hatred and bile on us with full force.

'Paki bastards! Little Paki bastards! Why don't you f-off home!'

'Shut up!' Zakir yelled back at them, angrily. 'Shut up! This is my home!'

All of a sudden one of them ran at him and punched him. An instant later the whole gang had set upon him. Like a pack of dogs they started hitting him and kicking him, screaming as they did so.

'Get him!'

'Get the Paki bastard!'

'Kick his Paki head in!'

For a second or so Zakir tried to fight back, and then he went down under a flurry of blows. He lay on the ground curled into a ball, trying desperately to protect his head with his arms. I screamed out and kept on screaming, as the pack of skinheads just kept kicking him over and over again. Luckily, Uncle

Kramat's son, Ahmed, heard me, and he raced to Zakir's aid. As more of the men on the street mobilised themselves, the skinheads saw the way things were going and fled.

Zakir was left lying on the ground, writhing in pain. I was terrified. How badly hurt was he? There was a stream of blood pouring out of his nose. When we tried to move him, it was clear that he was in agony. Most of the pain was around his ribs, where the skinheads had really been putting the boot in. Slowly and carefully, we helped pull Zakir to his feet. He was just about able to walk.

'You okay?' Ahmed asked. 'You want me to drive you to the hospital?'

'I'm fine,' replied Zakir, spitting out some blood. 'No fuss. I don't want any fuss. I just want to go home. Mum can clean me up.'

Zakir's nose looked broken and his lips were split and bleeding. He had the beginnings of a big black eye. Mum was horrified at what the 'goray lowlife' had done to him. After bathing Zakir's wounds, she went and told the local police officer, and he got the police to come and ask a few questions at the college. But nothing more was done. And no one on our street really wanted anything done, either.

Everyone just wanted the whole thing to go away. If anyone was arrested and tried, it would only serve to shine a light into our community. And that would be far from welcome. We kept ourselves to ourselves – that was the way on our street. The community knew about the attack within hours of it happening. And from that point on no one ever walked past the college alone. The skinheads must have realised that the whole community was on the lookout, for all they ever did was call names.

What had happened frightened me, but it didn't make me feel differently about white people. Most of my friends at school were white, and they stuck up for me. They were my champions. But it did make me feel differently about skinheads. I decided that that was just what skinheads were like. They were their own, closed tribe – a racist, ignorant one at that. In a sense, the skinhead tribe had similarities to my own: they lived by a set of rules informed by blind prejudice and ignorance.

At school I started getting called a 'Paki' and a 'Saddam-lover'. It was mainly some of the older boys who didn't know me. Most of the time I didn't respond. Sometimes, I tried to explain to them that Pakistan was not the same country as Iraq, and that the war was nothing to do with us. But they wouldn't listen. Luckily for me, Lara became my foremost champion – and which of the boys would ever want to offend the most beautiful girl in our year!

Lara was a lovely person, and fiercely loyal. When people tried to have a go at me or call me names, Lara would jump in to defend me.

'Leave her alone, you idiot!' she'd say, her eyes blazing furiously. 'She's nothing to do with it!'

'But she's a Paki . . .'

'Just shut up!' Lara would cut in. 'Duh! Pakistan. Iraq. Get the difference? Duh-brain!'

'But . . .'

'Look, you don't know *anything*. So before you say something even more stupid, best shut up. Don't you reckon?'

Lara knew how stupid they were to think that I had anything to do with the Gulf War. It was a war being fought on behalf of one Muslim country, Kuwait, against another Muslim country, Iraq. She was quite right in saying it was nothing to do with me.

'What's it got to do with Pakistan?' she'd declare, angrily. 'It's happening in Arabia! Don't suppose you know the difference, do you?'

The lads would pay attention to Lara for the simple reason that they all fancied her. The last thing they wanted was to look stupid and imbecilic in front of her. She was their dream girlfriend, and she was my greatest protector.

The teachers knew this was going on. They knew some of the white kids were causing trouble. My English teacher, Mrs Zorba, decided to have a class discussion about it, in an effort to defuse the tension. A couple of the most troublesome lads had brothers in the Army who had been sent to the Gulf to fight. They were angry about their brothers being put in harm's way. They didn't see why they should risk their lives on behalf of a distant country that no one had ever heard of. And they didn't see why they shouldn't vent some of their anger on the nearest brown Muslim – me.

Mrs Zorba's lesson gave me a chance to explain things from my point of view. I said that I thought people generally shouldn't go to war if they could possibly avoid it. And I explained that my community – the Pakistani Muslims – were entirely anti-Saddam, which largely we were.

My father was split on the war. He didn't support Saddam, because he was a secular leader. He had got rid of sharia law and other Islamic customs in Iraq, which didn't earn him my father's support. But at the same time he didn't like the fact that British soldiers were going to war in a Muslim country. He agreed there had to be an intervention to help the Kuwaitis, but argued it should come from the Saudis, or other Muslim countries.

The fact that few Muslim countries had militaries capable of taking on the Iraqi Army was ignored by my father. The fact that the war was sanctioned by the UN, and that the forces were an international coalition, also appeared lost on him.

'Look at them!' he'd declare angrily, when there were news reports on TV. 'Goray marching all over Muslim soil. They are taking over the Muslim lands!'

After the discussion in Mrs Zorba's class, things were easier for me at school. The lads seemed to understand that I was neutral on the war, and I understood why they felt so angry about it. They didn't want this war because their loved ones were in the firing line. I didn't want this war because I disagreed with war per se. So what was there to argue about? Soon, the bullying and name-calling dropped off almost to nothing.

Thanks to Lara, and Mrs Zorba, no one called me a 'Saddam-loving Paki' any more.

Everyone in Mrs Zorba's English class had to do a book review, which was to be presented in front of the class. I chose to review *To Kill a Mockingbird*, by Harper Lee. It tells the story of a white family in the American south, whose father, Atticus Finch, has to defend a black man falsely accused of raping a white girl. It is a classic tale of a principled man who champions justice in a seemingly hopeless situation. To me it was a passionate cry for tolerance, and the need to live and let live – the sort of message that my father, and the skinhead 'dolies' alike, had clearly never heard.

I tried to write a good review because I loved English, and because Mrs Zorba was my favourite teacher. Her name didn't sound English, but she looked like many other English people to me. She was tall and slim and she had to be somewhere in her mid-fifties. Her age showed in her face and hands, which were finely wrinkled. She had grey hair, which she wore in a bun, with wispy strands falling loose at the front.

Mrs Zorba was gentle and softly spoken, and it was with her that I found myself able to feed my love of reading. She was so supportive of me, and full of encouraging words. But when it came time to present my book review, I felt sick with nerves. Standing up in front of the class, I was shaking with fear. I went to start reading, but something just snapped.

I ran out of the classroom and ended up hiding in the girls' loo. I sat there for a while, crying my eyes out and feeling like a total failure. It wasn't until the lesson had finished that I managed to pull myself together enough to leave the loo. I went back to the classroom and found Mrs Zorba tidying up her books.

'I'm sorry I ran away,' I mumbled.

She smiled at me. 'That's all right. Are you feeling better?'

I nodded. 'A little.'

'Why did you run?' she asked.

'I was just so nervous . . . I was scared everyone would laugh at me and at what I wrote.'

'I tell you what. How about I read over your review? If *I* think it's good, would you be brave enough to present it then?'

'I'll try,' I said. But I was still terrified at the prospect.

Later that day Mrs Zorba came and found me in one of the corridors.

'I've read it,' she said. 'And you know what – it's really good. You really felt this story, didn't you?'

'I guess I did.'

'So, will you read it out in class like you promised?'

'I just don't think I can,' I stammered. 'I'm too scared. I don't want to.'

'Well, don't worry. I won't force you to. I just wanted you to know that it's good stuff.'

At the start of her next lesson Mrs Zorba stood up in front of the class.

'Thank you, everyone, for your work,' she announced. 'Now, I'm going to read you a really excellent book review, so you can see what we're aiming for. It's a review of *To Kill A Mockingbird*, by Harper Lee.'

The colour rose to my face, but thankfully Mrs Zorba didn't say it was my work. She just read it out, and then moved on with the lesson. I couldn't believe it. At home, no one had ever said that I was good at anything. All I was ever good enough for was graft, beatings and abuse. I was left with a warm glow of pride.

At the end of that year we received a letter at home announcing that I'd won the Bermford Comp prize for English. None of my brothers had ever won a school prize before. I was so proud, and my brothers seemed pretty chuffed, too. As for Sabina, she just did her best to ignore it. I read Mum the letter, and she seemed really pleased. But Dad just ignored it – as he did with me the whole time, unless he was abusing me.

By this time Zakir and Billy were both away at university. As for poor Raz, the madrassa was to be the sum total of his 'higher education'. The school prize-giving was to be held in the evening, and neither of my parents wanted to go. They wouldn't let me go on my own, and for a while it looked like I would miss it. But kindly Raz stepped in to help. His three years of hell in the madrassa hadn't knocked the heart out of him completely. He offered to act as my chaperone at the prize-giving.

'You know,' Raz remarked, as he walked me to school that

evening, 'you've done really well. You should feel good about yourself. This is your big day.'

I wanted to hug Raz, and tell him how grateful I was that he'd agreed to take me. But no one ever showed any sign of affection in our household, and we certainly never hugged. The only physical contact I ever had was sickening and obscene – my dad panting and pawing at me in the cellar.

The letter had told me that my prize was a cheque for £29, which I would get on the night. Beforehand, I had to buy books to that amount. I chose a Compact Oxford English Dictionary, which was the most expensive thing in the bookshop, plus a novel called *The Outsiders*. This had been my favourite book from the age of thirteen. I had read it over and over again.

It is about a gang of lads in America, three of whom are brothers. Their parents die in a car crash, and the eldest has to look after the younger two. The story is told from the perspective of the youngest. He and his best friend murder someone from another gang, and they have to go into hiding. Their gang of friends support them and shield them. The book is about the relationships between the gang members, and about how the main character feels about his parents.

Though our situations were superficially very different, I related to the main character very closely. Like me, he mostly hated his life. He was an outsider in his world, because he didn't like the gang or the gang culture. He had been forced into it, and there was no way out. He was wearing the 'skin' of a tough gang member and a murderer, even though in his heart he wasn't like that at all.

In that sense he was me: I wore the skin of a subservient Muslim girl and the Imam's daughter, whereas in reality I was dying inside and desperate to be free. I wasn't in a gang, but I was trapped in a culture that I neither liked nor related to. As I got older, I felt more and more alienated from my street. And I had to hide the abuse from everyone. I wore a skin, and I had to be a pretender. That was why *The Outsiders* spoke to me so powerfully.

With those two books my £29 was gone. The town's Mayor presented the prizes, handing me my books in front of the cameras. Those were the first books that I ever owned – apart from the Quran. They were utterly precious to me. I put them in my hiding place on top of the wardrobe.

I hoped that no one could find, steal or hurt them up there.

Chapter Thirteen

The English Prize

Unfortunately, the English prize was a bright moment in what was becoming a deteriorating school record for me. From the time that I had first worn Sonia's clothes, my spirit of rebellion grew and grew, and it began to manifest itself in increasingly erratic and troublesome behaviour at school.

One day we were in a classroom that had a walk-in storeroom off to one side. The teacher would go into it occasionally, to fetch books or other school supplies. I had noticed that there was a key in the door, and I had thought idly about locking someone in there.

We had a new teacher that day – a young, fresh-faced woman who had some difficulty in controlling the class. Towards the end of the lesson she went into the storeroom to fetch something. Quick as a flash and without even thinking, I jumped up, slammed the door, and locked it from the outside.

For a second everyone just stared at me in amazement, and then they burst out laughing. I had always been such a good and quiet student, and I was never in trouble. I could see people staring at me in surprise. *Wow! What a trick Hannan's pulled!* That's what they were all thinking. *Never knew she had it in her!*

At the same time I could hear the teacher inside the cupboard, shouting and banging on the door. I didn't know what on earth I had done, or what to do next. As time ticked away, I could hear the teacher getting more and more panicked. Just before the bell went for the end of class, I unlocked the door – and everyone ran out in a big crush so as to hide who was responsible.

The teacher hadn't caught me, and I knew no one would ever snitch. But at the start of her next class she announced that we would all be in detention, unless the person who had locked her in the cupboard owned up. I got up, and admitted what I'd done.

I wasn't particularly worried about owning up to it. I still thought it was quite funny, as did all my friends. I certainly didn't want anyone else getting into trouble. It would have stopped being a joke had all my friends got detention because of it. I alone was put in detention, and I had to write five hundred lines: *I will never lock my teacher in the cupboard again. I will never lock my teacher in the cupboard again.*

Mrs Zorba came to have a little talk with me about what I had done.

'I hear you locked your new teacher in the cupboard,' she remarked. 'That's not like you. What's going on?'

I didn't really know what to say, so I just shrugged. Even I didn't understand why I had done it. In fact, it was all about me rebelling in any way that I could, but I wasn't consciously aware of that yet. I had few opportunities to break out of the straitjacket of my life at home, so I seized upon anything that I could at school – like the key in the cupboard door. And of course, if I rebelled at home the fate that awaited me there was infinitely worse than writing a few lines.

Not long after that I started to play truant. There was an alleyway a couple of streets away from the school where those who had bunked off lessons hung out. The lads who played truant would generally catch a bus into the town centre, but the girls weren't so daring. So the alleyway was pretty much our domain.

It was hardly used by anyone else and relatively private, and there were steps on which you could sit and chat. There were rarely any boys to flirt with, but there were alcohol and cigarettes to be had. A shopkeeper around the corner was quite happy to sell us cheap bottles of cider, and single cigarettes at ten pence apiece – even though we were far too young to buy either legally.

Karen was the lead truant out of all of us. She had been truanting for ages, and her family didn't seem to care. Sometimes we'd go round to her house when bunking off lessons. If her parents were there they wouldn't mind. Karen was even allowed to smoke at home, and her parents gave her the cigarettes.

Karen and Amanda loved the thrill of smoking and drinking. One day I took a drag on a cigarette, but I didn't really like it. I tried drinking cider, but the taste was horrible. Of course, I knew that smoking and drinking were haram – forbidden – in my own culture and religion. And that was exactly the appeal for me. I was excited by the sense of rebellion, the power I suddenly possessed to defy my parents.

Normally, the class register would be taken first thing in the morning and last thing in the afternoon. Bunking off class in between was easy enough. But one day the school fire alarm went off. I was in the alleyway with Karen and Amanda and we didn't hear it ring – and so we weren't present when they took an extra register. Immediately, the teachers realised we were absent from school.

When the three of us reappeared at the end of the school day we were marched in front of the deputy head.

'Where were you?' he demanded. 'Why weren't you in class? We know you weren't at school. I hope you realise the trouble you're in.'

The deputy head didn't want answers. He knew we'd been bunking off class. He told us that this was our first warning. If we truanted again, we'd be before the headmaster. If we did it again, there would be detention every night for a week. After that, we'd have to take all our classes in a special truants' room. Following that, they'd write to our parents and suspend us for a few days. And if that didn't work, we'd be expelled from school.

I found an easy way around this. Because my parents couldn't read or write English, I had always written my own sick notes. I realised that there was nothing to stop me doing the same to cover my truanting. It wasn't as if my teachers could ring up my parents to check if they were genuine, for neither side could understand the other. Unlike Amanda and Karen, I had the perfect get-out-of-gaol-free card!

But increasingly, my problems weren't about being free to bunk off school – quite the reverse, in fact. I was growing ever more troubled by my dread of going home. I dreaded the domestic chores that I was forced to do, and I dreaded what Dad might do to me if I did anything to 'provoke' him. Whilst my friends wanted to bunk off school so as to spend more time at home, I wanted to bunk off home and remain at school.

Sometimes, I was so fearful of leaving that I would sit there at the end of school, refusing to go. I did this especially in Mrs Zorba's class, because I felt that I could trust her. Mrs Zorba would be packing her bag, or wiping off the blackboard, and I'd be sitting in the classroom. Eventually she'd glance up and find me alone at my desk.

'Hannan, you're still here?' she'd comment. 'No home to go to this evening?'

'There's a *home* all right,' I'd mutter. 'I just don't want to go there.'

'Why not?' she'd ask me, gently.

'It's horrible at home,' I'd mutter. 'I hate it there.'

Mrs Zorba would try to get me to explain myself. Eventually, I'd admit to her a small part of the reason why I didn't want to leave.

'I'm like the family servant. I have to do all the cooking, the cleaning, the laundry . . . I'm just so tired and fed up with it all.'

At times I broke down in tears as I talked to Mrs Zorba. She was very sweet and sympathetic. She would pass me a handkerchief to dry my eyes. But whilst she was trying to be helpful, she had little idea of what it was like living in my community, with my parents. She used to suggest that I try sitting down with my mum and dad, to have a little chat with them about what was wrong. *As if!*

I didn't want to tell her how naive and misguided her advice to me actually was. From her world-view it probably seemed perfectly sensible, but from mine it was dangerous nonsense. Any attempt at a frank discussion with my parents would just earn me another savage assault. My father's rage would know no bounds at my 'defiance', and the darkness would envelop me.

I told Mrs Zorba that I'd give her advice a try, but it was a lie. The more erratically I behaved, and the more I played truant, the more concerned she became for me. Finally, she realised that something had to be seriously wrong at home. I was hanging around in her lesson at the end of another school day when Mrs Zorba must have decided to grasp the nettle. She came and sat next to me.

'Hannan, I'm really worried about you,' she said. 'Something's really not right at home, is it? That's why you don't want to leave. Come on, why don't you tell me. I can't help you unless I know what's really the matter, can I?'

I started to cry. There was no way in the world that I could find it in myself to 'confess' about the abuse. What would she think of me if I did? She would be disgusted and appalled. My favourite teacher would surely want nothing more to do with dirty little me.

'My dad's not nice to me,' I sobbed. 'Sometimes he hits me.'

'I'm so sorry, Hannan, I'm so sorry,' Mrs Zorba comforted me. 'No parent should ever hurt a child. Is there anything else?'

I didn't say another word. What could I say? I just cried and cried.

'Look, Hannan, I want to talk to the deputy head about my concerns,' Mrs Zorba ventured. 'Is that okay with you?'

'No, it's not okay. Please don't tell anyone. *Please.*'

I didn't want Mrs Zorba saying anything to anyone, because I didn't want Dad to find out. If he had the slightest inkling that I might be spilling the beans on him, I dreaded to think what he might do. That was my greatest fear. As far as I was concerned, in my home, my family and my community my father was all-powerful. He was the head of the family and the untouchable Imam. How could I ever stand up to him?

Mrs Zorba gave a sigh. 'Hannan, I'm really sorry, but I have to say something. I'm not allowed to keep this quiet. It's my duty as your teacher to report something like this. If a pupil is this upset, it's a sign that she really does need help. I have to say something, especially if I think there might be a danger to you or others in your family.'

I couldn't tell her why I didn't want her to talk to anyone – *he'll drag me into the cellar* – yet at the same time I didn't seem able to stop her. That evening, as I made my nervous, fearful way home, Mrs Zorba was in the deputy head's office having words. She'd asked me to go with her but I had refused. The next day she told me what had transpired. They had decided that I needed to see a social worker.

I'm sure Mrs Zorba suspected there was more going on than just the physical violence. The signs were there for all to see, if only anyone had looked for them. And her words to me the previous evening had suggested as much. *Is there anything else, Hannan? Anything else . . .* All she could see was a terrified little girl afraid to go home to her violent father, and she suspected worse. She hoped I might open up further to a social worker, a professional. But the prospect frightened the life out of me.

'I can't talk to anyone else, Mrs Zorba! I'll get into trouble if I do. I just want to talk to you.'

'Hannan, listen – you won't get into trouble. So don't worry. These people are professionals, and it is your right to talk if you want to. They talk to teenagers all the time. They're used to keeping secrets. They are here to help. It'll be okay.'

With Mrs Zorba's words to calm me I agreed to go along with it. A week later I was told to go to the deputy head's office after lunch. The social worker would be waiting there to talk to me. I was so nervous I didn't dare tell any of my friends what was going on. I made my way to the deputy head's office, my feet dragging like lead.

As I waited outside I was shaking, and I felt almost physically sick. But there was a part of me that really wanted to talk to someone. I was desperate for a way out. Perhaps this was it? Perhaps I could finally unburden myself of all the dirt, guilt and shame? Perhaps the person listening – the social worker – would be able to help me?

I hadn't been waiting long when the deputy head came for me. He showed me into the consultation room.

'Hannan, this is your social worker,' he announced, pointing me in the direction of the lone figure standing by the window. 'His name is Omer.'

Instantly, I felt as if I had been punched hard in the stomach. I grabbed the desk to steady myself as my world went dark. I stared over in his direction. *Surely they couldn't have* . . . But they had: Omer, my social worker and my supposed saviour, was a fellow Pakistani Muslim.

I had known as soon as I'd heard the name, and his appearance just confirmed it for me. Omer came from my community, my tribe. I didn't recognise him personally, but I didn't need to. He was one of us, and that alone was enough to put the fear of God into me – or worse still, my father.

Omer was dressed in jeans and a denim shirt. He was tall, with a stubbly chin, and he looked to be in his early thirties. Superficially he appeared to be so Westernised.

He tried a smile. 'Hi. It's Hannan, isn't it? I'm Omer. I've come over from the South Bermford office to have a chat with you, okay?'

South Bermford. It was a suburb on the outskirts of town, which was close enough. Without a doubt, this man would know my father. I panicked. What should I do? Should I blurt out that it was all a big mistake? *There was nothing wrong at home. Nothing. The teachers had got it wrong. My home life was a joy, and I'd just been messing.*

Of course, I had been *expecting* a white person, or at least someone not from within my community. I hadn't for one moment thought that they might send a fellow Pakistani Muslim to speak with me, and one from the locality. What on earth had they been thinking? Had they thought it was a good idea to send someone from the same religion and culture as me, that it might make me feel more at home? In fact, the reverse was true. This was the worst possible scenario, and it terrified me.

One by one these thoughts bombarded me. I felt sick with worry. And then I became aware of Omer staring at me, oddly.

'Hannan? Hannan?' he prompted. 'Did you hear what I just said?'

I shook my head. 'No. Sorry. What?' I mumbled.

'I asked if you're feeling all right?' Omer repeated. 'You look terrible, white as a sheet. I'm not a scary ghost. I'm just a social worker. There's nothing to be scared of.'

There's *everything* to be scared of, I thought. But I didn't say anything.

'Your teachers said you've been having some trouble at home,' Omer prompted. That smile again. 'What kind of problems are they, Hannan?'

Omer tried to coax me into talking. He smiled so much and was so reassuring that eventually I began to relax a little. He asked me lots of questions, and seemed so sympathetic. Perhaps I was wrong to have judged him so harshly, I thought. There were many good people in our community. Perhaps I could talk to him in safety.

Omer asked me why I didn't want to go home at the end of the school day. I told him that my family made me do all the housework, as if I was a slave. I said I hated my life and my home. He asked me what I was scared of and why it was so hateful. I told him that my father was ultra-strict and conservative, and I confessed that I was scared that I would be sent back to Pakistan and forced into a marriage.

I suspected that I was being lined up to marry my first cousin on Mum's side. Recently, I'd been shown a photo of him. He was a peasant farmer from the village back in Pakistan. Mum had cracked a 'joke' that they'd decided I was going to marry him. I'd thought: *you may be joking now – but it's probably true.* Mum had gone on and on about what a handsome man he was, and what a perfect match we'd make. I had barely glanced at the photo.

In our community girls were supposed to be married off at the earliest possible age, before they were tempted into 'dishonouring' the family by falling in love. The very idea of marrying for love was the zenith of 'dishonour', because it meant by default that you must have had 'inappropriate relations' prior to marriage. You must have met the person and spent time with them to be able to fall in love. The 'honourable' way of doing things was to have no contact with the groom prior to the wedding.

Parents were so keen to get their daughters married off that they paid a dowry to the groom to take them off their hands. Often, the man would get a chunk of money, a young, virgin British bride, and a ticket to the United Kingdom into the bargain. He would live with the bride and her family while he learned English and tried to get a job. Normally, he would have zero qualifications and be illiterate. He would be practically unemployable, and fit only for manual labour. And this was seen by the parents as a 'good match', and it was all done for the sake of 'honour'.

In India and Pakistan there are even 'dowry killings'. If the bride's parents can't afford to pay the dowry they murder their daughter, rather than risk the family being 'dishonoured'. I had heard many such stories, and I told Omer about some of them, but he kept pressing me for more. Eventually, he found a chink in my armour and got to me.

'But why are you so *frightened*, Hannan? Your teacher tells me you're scared to go home. Is there something you're not telling me?'

'He . . . he hits me,' I mumbled.

'Your father? Your father's violent towards you? And that's how he forces you into doing things you don't want – like an arranged marriage? Is that it?'

I nodded. 'Yes. Pretty much.'

I didn't go into any more detail. We were running out of time, anyway. Omer had an hour for me, and it was all but exhausted.

'I'll come back next week, Hannan, so we can continue our chat,' Omer assured me. 'We can talk as much or as little as you like. So don't worry, okay?'

Talking about this – even in the limited way that I had – felt so strange. I didn't know how to feel, really. That afternoon I walked home from school lost in thought. Omer had seemed like a nice man, after all. Perhaps I would agree to see him again. I went into the kitchen. Mum told me to make some tea and coffee with biscuits, and take it into the front lounge for Dad, as he had a visitor.

I made up the tray as I had done a thousand times before. My mind elsewhere, I knocked and entered into the lounge. And there, sitting on the sofa next to Dad, was Omer the social worker. He caught sight of me and smiled. *That smile again.* He acted as if it was the most natural thing in the world for him to be sitting there deep in discussion with my father.

I felt my blood run cold. I was absolutely terrified. As I put the tray down my hands were shaking. I backed out of the room, stumbling over a rough edge of the carpet. I rushed upstairs in a total panic. What on earth could I do? Should I run away? But where would I go? Should I take the pills? Shove every last one of them down my neck and open my heart to sweet oblivion?

But perhaps I was overreacting. Perhaps Omer was still on my side. Perhaps he hadn't even mentioned talking to me. Perhaps he'd just dropped around saying it was a routine call from the Social Services. Perhaps he was just having a good sniff around, checking out my father. Perhaps his visit might even be good for me. There was always a chance.

I didn't have long to dwell on such thoughts. I heard a call from the bottom of the stairs. It was my father. I came down, with each step my legs shaking in fear. Dad was standing in the lounge, the expression on his face one of a long-suffering saint, with an aberrant daughter to deal with. Instantly I knew what had happened. Omer had told Dad all that I had said, and Dad was doing his best cuddly holy man act. He'd told Omer that I was lying, and Omer either believed him, or didn't give a damn.

'Hannan, I've told your father what you said,' Omer announced. 'He says there's no truth to it. He's assured me that he will discuss with you openly your options for marriage. And he's told me he would never dream of striking any of his daughters.'

I could hardly breathe, I was in such shock. This was my worst ever nightmare. I was incapable of speaking a word. What was there that was worth saying? Omer and my father, two Muslim men of Pakistani origin, had done a deal. This was the worst ever betrayal.

Omer turned to my father. 'As far as I'm concerned, that's the end of the matter. I'm sorry to have troubled you, sir. I'm sure she's a good girl at heart.'

It was all so transparent. All Omer could think was how to protect my father, the Imam, and the honour of the community. In terms of protecting me, he just didn't care. Omer shook hands with my father, turned and gave me that smile again, and then he stepped out of the lounge. Dad showed him to the door.

An instant later he was back in again. He simply went berserk. He drew back his hand and punched me in the chest, and then he did it again. The second blow knocked me to the ground, but even then he had no mercy. He beat me up there and then, in the front lounge, raining down savage kicks and punches upon me.

There was nothing that I could do but take it. I curled into a ball, trying to protect myself. Mum was in the kitchen, and I guessed she could hear what was going on. But it didn't matter, anyway. I knew she would do nothing to intervene. Once again, I was utterly on my own.

'If you ever, *ever* breathe a word to anyone else, I'll kill you!' he hissed, his face a mask of utter evil. 'I'll kill you, and I'll enjoy doing it. You stupid, stupid, stupid, cursed, worthless, evil girl!'

He grabbed me by my hair, and dragged me through the kitchen. He threw open the cellar door and shoved me headlong down the stairs. I hit the ground with a hollow thump, landing in an agonised heap on the hard brick floor. I knew what was coming, and I begged him not to. But an instant later he was over me, ripping off my clothes. There, in the dark, he stripped me naked, beat and kicked my body, and raped me.

With a final, animal grunt he was finished with me. He climbed off my crushed body. But it wasn't over yet. In the corner was a dirty cord. Dad grabbed it, and tied it tight around my ankles and my wrists. As he pulled on it, it dragged my arms and legs backwards, forcing my body into a horribly contorted U-shape. Trussed up like that it felt as if my arms were about to be ripped from their sockets.

It wasn't the first time that my father had tied me. Now that I was a teenager, he wasn't able to cause me the same pain simply by raping me. The rope was his answer, his way to ensure that I'd be hurt, and be left in agony for hours and hours. I bit hard on my lip and tried not to scream, tasting the blood. I didn't want him to see my pain.

My eyes watered with tears, but I fought them back. I choked down the sobs. I knew he'd just enjoy it all the more, the more he knew he was causing me pain. When he tired of the torture, my father clambered back up the creaking wooden stairs. There was a momentary flash of brightness from the opening door. It swept the darkened cellar like a searchlight, and then the door slammed shut. I heard the key turn in the lock, and then all was silent, and I was left alone and drowning in the darkness.

I begged for the Loneliness Birds to come for me. Suddenly there was a bright flash of golden sunlight, and an eager fluttering above me. There they were! There were my beloved white doves. They had come to the rescue, to carry me out of that place of horror and dirt, and off to my clean, bright, dreamy place of rest – the Lavender Fields.

I came back to my senses a while later. I was covered in cuts and bruises, and I was in agony from the ropes. Every part of me ached, but most of all my heart and soul. As always, Dad had been very clever. He had not once hit me on the face. Instead, he had gone for my chest, back and legs. Under my shalwar kamiz no one would be able to see the damage he had inflicted upon me, the blue-yellow bruising that was spreading over my burning skin.

In fact, no one would see anything of me for a while now. My father left me locked in the cellar for days on end, even though it was term time and I was supposed to be at school.

Occasionally, Mum would bang on the cellar door with a plate of curry for me. She'd hand it over with downcast eyes, and not a word. As soon as I'd taken it she'd turn her head away and go back to her cooking or washing. Mum just didn't want to know. She was determined to ignore the reality of what her husband, the Imam, had become, and the dark, unspeakable evil lurking at the heart of her family.

As I languished in the cellar I realised that there was no way out. I had made my cry for help, and I had been sent first Omer, and now this. I thought more and more about taking those pills. If I was going to live, the only way to survive was to shut up completely. I would have to stop lingering behind at school. There was no point now, and it was dangerous. If it ended up with that bastard social worker being called in, and him reporting back to Dad, then I was caught in a never-ending nightmare.

I knew that my teachers had thought they were doing the best for me. Due to their 'cultural sensitivity' they had brought in someone from my own community to 'help' – presuming he would better be able to understand. What they didn't realise was that it was only someone from another tribe – from *outside* of my own community – who could offer me the help, and sanctuary, that I so desperately needed.

I didn't blame Mrs Zorba, or the deputy head. I blamed Omer, and with a vengeance. Once I was released from the hell of the cellar I would tell Mrs Zorba that I didn't ever want to see him again. I had made my cry for help, and as a result I had been thrust into betrayal and darkness. It was time to shut up and survive. Either that, or the pills.

A week later I was back at school, and who should I see in the corridor but Omer.

'Hannan!' he called out. 'We were supposed to meet. How about it? I've got a free hour this afternoon.'

I shook my head. 'No thanks.'

'No? Why not? Don't you want to talk some more?'

I looked him in the eye. 'No, I don't. And you're a real bastard, that's why.'

I could see the shock on his face. 'Hey, I was just doing what I thought was right – you know that. It's not right to betray your community . . .'

'Don't you ever come near me again!' I cut in. 'You know what – you're shit at your job. You know that? Totally shit.'

I wasn't about to wait for a reply. I turned my back and walked off. For people like him the honour of the community was always more important than the rights of any individual, even when that individual was a child. And that was the great trap of our culture that the white English teachers just didn't get. They had thought they were being 'culturally sensitive' by calling in an Asian social worker to talk to me.

In fact, they were driving me further into the hands of my abusers.

Chapter Fourteen

Dirty Little Me

I was fifteen, and my GCSEs were fast approaching. I was also becoming ever more desperate. I hated my home life. I was totally alienated from my family. I was rebelling against my culture, and my faith. I lived for my school days – my slice of freedom in a life that was enchained. Yet I knew for sure that sometime soon my education would come to an abrupt and bitter end.

I knew that my father was setting up an arranged marriage for me. Once I'd done my GCSEs, I'd be shipped off to that cousin in Pakistan. Problem solved. My life would be over, and Dad's rebel daughter would be long gone. The same had happened to a lot of girls on our street. In the summer holidays, after finishing their GCSEs, they would simply disappear. And we'd never hear from them again.

But there was another, darker factor at play with my family. As far as Dad was concerned, it was the perfect way to bury forever his abuse of me. I would never dare complain about what he had done to me once I was safely locked away in my 'husband's' house in rural Pakistan. I would be silenced, and he would get away with it. And as for Mum, the darkness at the heart of her family would finally be expunged. She could call a halt to her wilful ignorance, and unburden herself of the guilt.

No mention was being made by my parents of any marriage, but I felt certain that plans were quietly being laid. I wasn't doing that well at school, and Mum and Dad had already told me that I wasn't going to university. Pakistani girls didn't go to university, they said. Only boys went. I didn't argue with them. How could I? I just kept quiet, and hoped that somehow things might change.

At around this time, there was a story on the news about a British girl who had been taken to Pakistan and forced into a marriage. She had managed to get help from the British High Commission, and escaped. It was big news, and everyone had heard about it. My school friends were absolutely horrified.

'My God, it's so awful!' said Lara. 'How can you get married to someone you don't even know? Someone you don't love? Just imagine it! Yuk! Horrible!'

'I don't have to imagine it,' I remarked, quietly. 'It happened to my friend, Skip.'

Lara couldn't believe it. 'What? Who? Here in town? Or in Pakistan?'

'Here,' I said. 'She lived on my street. Then they sent her to Pakistan for a "holiday", and forced her to get married.'

'But how could a mum and dad do that to their daughter?' Lara asked. 'And why didn't she just tell them to get lost?'

'It's part of our culture,' I replied, bitterly. 'They do it to maintain the family's "honour". That's far more important than their daughter being happy.'

'Oh my God . . . Is that what's going to happen to you? Tell me it's not!'

I shrugged. 'Yeah, probably. I don't know, but it probably will. And it probably won't be long now . . .'

'But you can't!' Lara blurted out. 'You can't just go along with it. You've got to do something. Talk to your parents! Tell them you don't want to!'

I sighed. 'Look, Lara, you don't understand. There's no point talking to them. It'll only make it worse.'

It was inconceivable to Lara and my other white friends that their parents would do something like that to them. They had learnt in RE lessons about how Asian people got married with a dowry, and how it was often an arranged marriage. So in theory there was a kind of acceptance. But this was different. This was me. Lara was confronted by one of her best friends about to suffer the hell of a forced marriage, and it really brought the unspeakable injustice of it home to her.

Very little of our politically correct RE lessons had covered the dark and misogynistic side to arranged marriages. It was painted as a cultural and religious practice that, whilst seeming strange to most British people, should be treated with respect and understanding. The reality – that this so often constituted a shocking and brutal abuse of a woman's most basic rights – was hidden behind a smoke screen of political correctness.

As far as I was concerned, if two people wanted an arranged marriage that was fine by me. But a *forced* marriage was a very different thing. I had heard stories of Pakistani women running away from forced and abusive marriages, but because this was a 'shame' on their husband's honour, they had to go into hiding. If the husband or his family – *or even their own family* – caught them, they would be killed. In this warped mindset, a daughter's murder was far preferable to 'dishonour'.

I'd seen how Skip – spirited rebel Skip – had been drawn into a trap, and the miracle of her escape. I just knew that my dad was scheming, and that the next step in my betrayal was coming. Subconsciously, I decided to push things to the limit, to provoke a confrontation – to push at the frontiers of my own rebellion.

I had been wearing my friend Sonia's clothes on non-uniform days for a couple of years now. I had become quite relaxed about doing so. One day, I decided on the spur of the moment to walk down our street in my non-uniform get-up – jeans, T-shirt and no hijab. A lot of people saw me, and recognised me. I could see the shock and consternation on their faces. I felt a thrill of rebellion, and also a shudder of fear.

Unsurprisingly, someone went straight to my father and told him what they had seen. Once I'd changed my clothes at Sonia's house, I went home. There, I was confronted by Dad's towering rage.

'What were you doing?' he screamed as soon as he saw me. He grabbed me by the hair, twisting it savagely. 'Goray clothes! Becoming like "them"!'

He started to beat me. 'Flesh! Showing your bare flesh! Showing flesh like a gori whore!'

By now, Zakir was a grown man, and he was physically as strong as my father. It was a Friday, and I knew that he was home from college. There was no way that he couldn't hear my father's screaming, or the blows. But no one intervened, even when my father started dragging me towards the cellar.

Whenever Dad raped me, he made sure to couple it with violence. In that way it could be dressed up as 'punishment', rather than what it was – him satisfying his sick and evil sexual desires. I was locked in the cellar through to the Monday, missing yet another day of school whilst I languished in my dark prison.

When I was released I didn't appeal to my brothers for help. I didn't have that sort of relationship with them. Over the past year I had cut myself off more and more from my family. I felt more comfortable at school with my friends around me, in an environment where there was no chance of being beaten or sexually abused. I felt like an alien in my own home, and always in danger.

I was haunted by my past, terrified by the present, and fearful of the future. I was disturbed. My behaviour began to deteriorate rapidly. Where once I'd been a model student, now I was withdrawn, underachieving, and sometimes even violent.

One day I was on the bus with Sabina, my goody-goody sister, when another Pakistani girl, Sameena, started bullying her. Sameena was very Westernised, and she wasn't taken with Sabina's traditional dress – her shalwar kamiz and hijab.

'You're a real Paki,' she said with contempt. 'Why d'you dress like that? Why can't you look like the rest of us? You're a joke.'

I glanced at Sabina. She wasn't saying a word. I wondered why she couldn't, or wouldn't, stick up for herself.

Sameena carried on: 'You look so dumb! Why d'you have to show up the rest of us?'

I got up and went over to her. 'I've had enough of you calling my sister names,' I said. 'If you don't stop, I'm going to get you.'

Sameena laughed. 'You! You should tell her what's what! Your sister looks like a Paki from the village. Her clothes are hideous. Look at her with that stupid veil.'

Before I knew what I was doing, I felt my fist connect with her face. I had punched her. It was an astonishing moment. The last time I had stood up for someone was when I had shouted at Dad for beating Mum, and that was ten years ago. Sameena came back at me pulling my hair, and she raked her long nails across my cheek. They drew bright gashes of red, but I fought back hard. The two of us scrapped all the way to school. No one could stop us. When we got there, the teachers were called to break up the fight.

We were sent to our classes in disgrace. Later, we had to go and see the deputy head. Sameena and I stood before him as we were given a severe dressing-down. We were given a lunchtime detention and lines: *I must not fight on the bus. I must not fight on the bus. I must not fight on the bus . . .*

But it didn't seem to have any effect on Sameena. She continued to try to bully my sister, and so I continued to fight her. As for Sabina, she hated the fact that I was sticking up for her.

'You're just making it worse,' she told me. 'And, anyway, you're getting into trouble.'

I kept getting more detentions and punishments. But as far as I was concerned, Sameena had to be stopped. Sabina was repressed, and she never really stuck up for herself. I felt she needed a champion, even though she said she didn't. The first few times I fought with Sameena, my friends backed me up. But when I kept picking fights with her, they began to think it was too much.

'Let it go, Hannan,' Lara told me. 'Or report it to the teachers, so they can take some proper action. You can't keep dealing with it yourself. You'll just get into trouble.'

But I couldn't stop. I was obsessed with getting Sameena. It had become a real vendetta. We were fairly evenly matched. Her nails would often leave me bleeding, and a couple of times I managed to give her a black eye. But we always ended up being broken up by the teachers, so there was no decisive battle. For several months this went on. We'd have a big fight once a month at least. It was hugely disruptive to my studies, and no doubt to hers as well.

Eventually, I was hauled in front of the school head. 'Why are you fighting?' he asked. 'What's going on? Why do you and Sameena hate each other so much?'

At first I wouldn't talk. But in the end he got it out of me. 'She's bullying my sister. She calls her a "Paki". She says she wears stupid clothes.'

The head called in Sameena, and my sister, to ask them whether what I had said was true. Sabina said that it was, and gave them examples of the many occasions on which Sameena had bullied her. Sameena was suspended, and that was the end of the war between us.

For me, it had been to some extent a surrogate fight. I had never been able to stand up for myself at home, so I was trying instead to stand up for Sabina. All that pent-up rage that should have been directed at Dad had found its way into vicious fights with Sameena. She had behaved badly, there was no doubt about that. But for me this was much more about channelling my suppressed rage and anger into a violent release. Sameena had just presented a convenient target.

My English teacher, Mrs Zorba, could see the pain and confusion that possessed me. One day she spoke to me about it.

'Hannan, I know you're having trouble explaining why you're feeling the way you are,' she said. 'Why don't you try writing an essay for me? Treat it like a normal English assignment. Just write down anything that's bothering you.'

I called my essay: 'Asian Girls in Britain.'

When you are a teenager your parents watch you so closely and you have hardly any freedom. You start hating them, because they make you do horrid things you don't want. They make you do all the housework, even though you can't stand it. They want the traditions to carry on. They don't want to change how they live. You can't talk to them any more, because they can punish you by taking away what little freedom you have. The only freedom you have is at school, but they can stop you going anytime, even though it is against the law. You despise your brothers, because they have more opportunities than you. You have to wait on them hand and foot, like they're kings. You dread leaving school, because life will come to an end. You will lose all your freedom. The thought of running away goes through your mind each and every day.

Mrs Zorba gave my essay a top mark. But once she'd read it and realised how troubled I was, she tried again to find a way to help me. Would I see the social worker again, she asked. I told her I'd rather die. And that was pretty much the end of the matter. There wasn't much more that Mrs Zorba could do.

As my sixteenth birthday approached, my fears grew stronger and stronger. One day, Sabina found some passport application papers lying around on the table. They had been made out in my name. She told me all about it. Since I had stuck up for her at school, she had become slightly more friendly towards her big sister. It didn't stop her teasing me, though.

'Dad's going to ship you off to Pakistan,' she taunted. 'Hope you're looking forward to it! Soon you'll be off to meet your Paki lover . . .'

She wasn't being vindictive. She was just a little kid teasing her older sister. Sabina was so different from me. She was proud to conform, and she loved her traditional dress. She was looking forward to having a marriage arranged for her. Sabina used to say that she would happily go and live in Pakistan. There was an unbridgeable gulf between us.

I didn't say much when she taunted me over my 'Paki lover'. I wasn't really surprised. I'd known it was going to happen for a long time now. I also knew that I'd try to fight against it, but I didn't know exactly how. I still had those pills hoarded in my room. There was paracetamol, aspirin, and anything else that I had been able to get my hands on. If nothing else, having them in reserve gave me a dark and bitter strength.

Little did Sabina appreciate my fear of a forced marriage, or what I would do to avoid one.

Chapter Fifteen

Shackled Bride

My sixteenth birthday was in May that year. It wasn't a happy time for me. In fact, I was close to suicidal. I took my GCSEs, and already I knew that I hadn't done well. I reckoned my results would be appalling, and that Dad would use that as the final excuse to pack me off to Pakistan.

Sure enough, my results were abysmal. My best grade was a B in English. Other than that, I had two Cs, and the rest were all D and E. What a disaster. But it was hardly unexpected. My last year at school had been one of truanting, fighting and increasingly errant behaviour. There had been little study.

Still, I went ahead and applied to a Sixth Form College to do re-sits. I did so without my parents' knowledge. That summer there would be an induction day, and I really wanted to go and see what I might be able to study. With results like mine, the options would be painfully limited, but even so I lived in hope. I asked Mum whether I could take the morning off from house-work and go. To my surprise, she said yes. I don't think she even mentioned it to Dad.

It turned out that I needed four GCSE between A and C to go on and do A-levels, so that was out. But I could do re-sits. I decided that's what I would do, with a view to taking maths, RE, sociology, and business studies at A-level. Of course, I got the shock of my life when in due course Dad actually agreed to me going to the college. It was as if he didn't really care one way or the other. I wondered what was going on.

I couldn't quite believe it when that September came around, and I started my first day at South Bermford Sixth Form College.

I had been so convinced that by now I would be shackled to my 'husband' in Pakistan. Sabina had even told me that she'd overheard my parents discussing plans for my marriage. Yet still they had allowed me to go to college. Did this mean that I was in the clear for another two years? Or did they just want me to be doing something to occupy my time, while they put in place the final plans? I just didn't know.

I was the only one of my friends from secondary school who went on to further education. Lara and Amanda went to Bermford Technical College, to learn secretarial skills, cooking, childcare, and other 'vocational' skills. Karen had gone straight into working as a sales girl on a shop floor.

On that first day at college I met the lecturer who would become my favourite – Mrs Jones. Mrs. Jones taught Religious Studies. She was in her early forties, very tall and willowy, with sandy hair cut short and fashionable. She was very smartly dressed, and I was immediately struck by her presence, and her mature beauty.

Mrs Jones was a very caring person, with a big heart. She talked openly about her family in class. She would start each lesson with an informal chat about what was going on in her life, telling personal stories that helped illustrate the lesson.

Mrs Jones doubled as the school counsellor, and I had been at college for a month or so when I decided to go and see her for a chat. I wanted to talk to someone about my fears of an impending forced marriage.

'Miss, I'm really scared,' I told her. 'I know they're planning to marry me off, and send me to Pakistan. I don't want to go.'

'You poor thing,' Mrs Jones comforted me. 'I have to say I've heard such things before. I've had other girls come to me. Sadly, this sort of thing isn't news to me at all. Have you talked to your parents about how you feel? Can you?'

'No way,' I replied. 'Dad's the local Imam, and my family's very closed and strict. Talking won't help. In fact, it'll make it worse.'

'Well, I'm always here to talk, if you need me. But perhaps if you study hard, and get good grades, your parents might see that you should stay at college. These forced marriages are becoming a real problem, you know. The college is trying to work out how to deal with it. We are listening, Hannan, and we are here to help you.'

As I sat and talked to Mrs Jones, I realised that she was the 'Mrs Zorba' of the College – only she had much more experience of the problems faced by teenage girls in our community. I felt better having talked with her. I felt she really understood me. And I had felt safe in her room and in her presence. I had never felt this safe in my life before. But I still couldn't look at her. I couldn't make eye contact with any adults. Instead, I'd look at the floor or the wall – anywhere but directly at them. In a way, I talked and acted like a twelve year old, especially in terms of how shy and timid I was.

At the end of our conversation Mrs Jones said to me: 'I know I shouldn't say this, as you are a Muslim – but God really loves you, you know.'

'God loves me!' I just laughed. 'I'll believe it when I see it.'

God loves me? My father's god was incapable of loving anyone. My father's god was a cruel, avenging one that laughed at my misfortune. My father's god sat in harsh judgement, and had already condemned me to hell. So said my father, the Imam, in the same breath as telling me that *he* was going to heaven. And as far as I was concerned if Dad was the sort of person you found in heaven, I didn't want anything to do with his god, and I definitely didn't want to end up there.

That first time I went to see Mrs Jones I told her about my fears of an arranged marriage, and all about my dreams of going to university and living a life that was free. The second time I went to see her, she asked me if I wanted to see a social worker. At first I said no. No way. No way did I want a re-run of the nightmare I'd had with Omer, the betrayer. But eventually, she talked me around.

I agreed to see one as long as they weren't Asian. That was my one condition. I didn't explain why that was so, and Mrs Jones didn't ask. She just seemed to understand.

A few days later Barry turned up at college. He was a white guy in his late thirties, small and stocky with a big moustache. He was dressed in a suit and an open-necked shirt. The feeling I got from him was a warm and caring one. His eyes were gentle when he spoke, and I instinctively felt I could trust him. He had a great big smile, and it was genuine.

Barry never once spoke to me about honour or shame, or my family's reputation. He just wanted to hear about my own, personal fears and worries. He wanted me to talk all about me – freely, and stripped of any religious or cultural constraints. I saw Barry several times, and the bond of trust between us grew and grew. Eventually, Barry gave me a black and white guarantee of help.

'Hannan, if you ever feel that your parents are going to make you do anything against your will, or if you ever feel in danger, you can tell me and I will help you. I'll sort it out. There are ways in this country to really, really protect you.'

They were kind words, and perhaps a promise of the salvation I had only ever been able to dream of. But I wondered if he really could do all that he said. After all, Barry was from outside my community. Within it, Dad had far more power than he did. My father the Imam was the most powerful person in my life, and that was all I knew.

I knew my dad could ship me off to Pakistan. I knew my family and the community would close ranks and back him. It was what they *expected* to happen. It was what they *approved* of. It was what most were planning to do with their own daughters. If anyone ever came to investigate my disappearance, they would throw up a wall of lies and silence. Everyone would say that I had gone off willingly and was happy with my new life in Pakistan.

Barry also talked about my lack of confidence, and how I might build it up. He got me to write a list of things that others might find to like about me, and what I liked about myself. And he helped me practise looking at him while I talked, and making eye contact.

I found Barry's exercises really helpful. I realised that I could communicate so much more effectively when I actually looked at someone. What was more, I understood Barry better when I looked at his face and his expressions. I tried it with my teachers. Their response to me – their facial expressions, and their ability to relate to me better – helped me build my confidence further. It was a virtuous circle.

In my final year at secondary school my attitude had been awful. At college it improved tremendously. Maybe Mrs Jones was right, I thought. Maybe study and academic achievement were a way out. If I studied hard and did well, maybe my parents would let me go to university. I began to work harder than I ever had in my life before.

I didn't talk about any of this at home, but still I lived in hope. It was a hope that Mrs Jones had given me. In October, Mrs Jones suggested that the college send an ad hoc report to my parents, telling them how well I had been doing.

'Do you think it might help?' she asked me.

'It can't do any harm. It's worth a try.'

A few days later I took that report home with me. It looked so smart, with the college emblem proudly displayed on the front. My parents still couldn't read any English, so I had to read it for them, translating it into Punjabi as I did so. This is what it said:

Hannan has been working very hard, and the results of that hard work are becoming clear. She shows great promise. In recent Mathematics and Religious Studies tests, she achieved excellent marks and was placed high in the class. In both cases, she also achieved an A for effort. She is a pleasure to teach.

I could tell Mum was pleased. 'Well done!' she smiled.

Dad snorted. 'Oh well. That's that then.'

That was all the comment he ever made about it. It was never discussed again. I kept the report for myself. I wasn't overly disappointed. Part of me had been expecting just that kind of reaction from Dad.

Two weeks later I was at home doing my evening chores. I walked past the living-room door and heard someone speaking on the telephone. It was my father. Something made me stop and listen. I pressed my ear to the door.

'Yes, yes – we'll be flying out the day after tomorrow, arriving Karachi the afternoon. You'll be there to meet us, is it? Good. Is all set for the wedding . . . ?'

Oh my God, it was happening!

Somehow, I'd convinced myself that Sabina was wrong, that there were no secret wedding plans afoot. I had started to believe that there might be a way out via my studies. As far as I knew I didn't even have a passport. *So how could this be happening?*

Knowing how rebellious I had become, Dad was putting in place the final details of my marriage. Allowing me to go to college had been a total sham. It was just a trick designed to control me for long enough to get me shipped me off to Pakistan. Once I was there in the tribal areas and married to a distant relative, there would be no way back to the corrupting influences of Britain. Dad's problem – his eldest daughter – would have been dealt with.

For the past few months I had lived in false hope and with a false sense of security. Now I knew different. I knew that my abduction was planned and ready for the very next day. I would be bundled onto a flight in the evening, after college finished, overnight to Pakistan. And I would have my hated father by my side.

I ran upstairs to the bedroom. I was hyperventilating. I was beside myself with panic. I knew that I had to escape, but how? All I could think of was going to college the following day as if all were normal.

And then I would never come home again.

Chapter Sixteen

Honour and Shame

The phone was kept in the living room, but there was also a phone socket in our bedroom. Quite often, my brothers would take the handset upstairs to talk in private. I waited until Dad had left the house, then I crept down, took the phone and plugged it in upstairs. Everyone else was in the lounge watching TV.

I dialled Skip's number. I was scared stiff of being overheard, but I had to do something. One of my sisters or Mum could walk in at any time. Mum wouldn't understand all that I was saying in English, but she was sure to get the drift of it. Even she couldn't miss words like 'wedding' and 'Pakistan'. My sisters would know immediately, and I knew for sure that Sabina would tell my parents.

The phone rang and rang. For a second I feared that Skip wasn't going to answer. Then a voice.

'Hello?'

'Skip? Skip! It's Hannan. It's happening tomorrow night. The wedding! They've already got me a passport and a plane ticket. I'm so scared!'

'Oh my God! Right, let's think. It's tomorrow night, after college, is it?'

'After college – the overnight flight to Karachi.'

'Then you've got to leave right now.'

'I can't! I'm not allowed out at night. Especially alone. Anyway, where would I go?'

'All right, all right . . . Well then you've got to get out tomorrow morning, or you'll be trapped. Leave for college and that's it. I'll come and pick you up after college in my car, okay?'

'Okay.'

'I'll be waiting for you somewhere near the gates. You know the car, so as soon as you see it jump in.'

Skip was working as a secretary in an office, which meant she had enough money to buy her own car. But she was temporarily living back at home, as the lease on her flat had run out. She was dying to get away again. It was actually better for her family – less 'shameful' – to have an unmarried daughter living at home. That's why her parents had taken her in again. Just as soon as she could, she was going to get her own place. But for now it meant that I couldn't stay with her.

'Where will I go?' I said.

'I don't know. We'll sort something out. Worst comes to the worst, you can sleep in my car. Anything's better than your father taking you to bloody Pakistan!'

I didn't sleep a wink that night. I was gripped by anxiety, and a dark fear and trepidation. But I never for one moment lost heart. This was it – do or die. I had to get away. I had to escape. The cogs were whirring round in my head as I ran through Skip's plan, trying to spot any snags. I couldn't afford to make a mistake the next day. I only had the one chance.

I tried to get up at the normal time. I tried to keep everything just as it always was. I made everyone breakfast, but I was jumping with nerves. I packed my school bag, hiding a pair of jeans that Sonia had given me beneath some files. Then I was ready. I walked out of the front door, saying goodbye to my little sister, Aliya, for perhaps the last time. I tried to keep my voice normal. I was struggling to control the wild mixture of emotions that I was feeling.

I walked up our street knowing that I was never coming back. But at the same time I had no idea where I might end up. I couldn't go to any of my friends that lived on the street, obviously. Their parents would simply call my dad. I didn't know if the college tutors could help me, either, but I had to try. And there was always the promise that had been made to me by Barry, the social worker. If there was ever a moment when he needed to come good on it, now was the time.

I arrived at my first lesson five minutes late. For a second I just stood at the back and stared at the lecturer, Mrs Smith, a white lady in her thirties. She knew about my problems because of what Mrs Jones had told the college board. All of a sudden I just found myself yelling at the top of my voice.

'I've run away! I'm never going back! Never! Never going home . . . No matter what anyone says!'

The class was pretty full. Everyone turned around to stare at me. I could see the worry on their faces. Normally I was shy and quiet, and hardly attracted any notice. Now I was close to hysterical. They knew something was wrong, but none of them understood what I was going on about. Thankfully, Mrs Smith did.

She came over to me. 'Okay, Hannan, it's okay . . . We'll sort everything out. Don't worry. Just calm down.'

She told the class to occupy themselves for five minutes, whilst she took me to the principal's office. There was no one there, but she put me in a chair and told me to wait.

'I'll call Mrs Jones and your social worker,' she assured me. 'But for now just take it easy. They'll be with you soon, okay?'

A few minutes later Mrs Jones turned up, and shortly after that there was Barry. I blurted out all that had happened.

'My dad was on the phone last night and I heard him and it's all arranged for this evening and they're flying me out to Pakistan for an arranged marriage and I'm not going and there's no way I can go home tonight! No way!'

Barry glanced at Mrs Jones. 'Right. Well, first off – don't worry. We'll just have to find you somewhere safe to stay. I'll get on to it right away. You have my office number? Right, give me a call once you've finished college, and I'll have it sorted. It's nothing to worry about, okay? You're safe with us.'

I didn't know if Barry had the power or resources to find me somewhere just like that. But I was convinced he would try. In any case, I knew that I wasn't going home. If I had to I would sleep in Skip's car like she had said. It was a bitterly cold November, and it wasn't exactly an appealing option. I was scared and alone, and I didn't want to spend my first night as a runaway sleeping in my friend's car. But I wasn't going home.

At the end of the college day I was still unsure of what was going to happen. I sneaked out of the college gates, and my heart leapt with joy. There was Skip in her little blue car! She waved at me. I rushed over and jumped in, and told her everything that had happened.

We drove into the centre of town, and when we got close to Barry's office I stopped to use a payphone. I was uncertain and fearful, and I was dead scared in case any of my family spotted me. And I still had no idea whether Barry had found me anywhere. But just as soon as I heard his voice I knew that he'd managed it.

'I've got somewhere,' he announced. 'Everything's okay. Come and meet me at my office and I'll take you there right away.'

My heart skipped with hope. Skip gave me a hug. She drove me round the corner to his office and delivered me into Barry's care, wishing me good luck.

'I've found you somewhere safe,' Barry told me as he took me to his car. 'It's a short drive away. Come on!'

We set off across town. Soon, I realised that we were going to pass by the end of my street, and, for an instant, fear flashed before me. For one, awful moment I thought maybe Barry was going to do the same thing as Omer – deliver me back into the hands of my abusers. But a moment later we shot past and continued to the outskirts of town, some twenty minutes' drive away.

We stopped in front of a large, detached, brick-built house, with a lawn at the front. Barry went and knocked on the door. For a few seconds we waited, and then who should appear but my Religious Studies teacher, Mrs Jones! I was completely dumbfounded.

'Welcome, Hannan!' she declared, with a wonderful smile. 'I'm so glad you're here. Come on in.'

Barry and I were taken into the front lounge. Mrs Jones shut her two Jack Russell dogs in the kitchen, so they wouldn't jump all over us, and gave us tea and biscuits. I sat there holding tightly to my school bag, feeling nervous and uncomfortable. For my whole life I had dreamed about running away and escaping my family. Now I was finally doing it. I hadn't had time to think or process anything. The shock was starting to overwhelm me.

'After we spoke to you Barry and I had a chat,' Mrs Jones explained. 'Now, I've got a spare room. And my husband and I are very happy for you to stay here, if you're happy to. What d'you think, Hannan? Would you like to stay with us for a while?'

I didn't say very much. I just smiled weakly. I hadn't realised that she was actually going to let me stay *here*, in her family home. I'd presumed that Barry and I were stopping by on our way to somewhere else. I was drifting into shock, and I was terrified that my family would find out where I was and come and get me. I thought Dad was more powerful than anyone – the social worker, teachers, whoever. I was convinced that he would find out where I was, and drag me back again.

It was six o'clock by now, and my family probably had still to realise that I'd done a runner. I could easily have been walking home from college with friends. My flight to Karachi wasn't scheduled until close to midnight, so they wouldn't be panicking just yet. But that didn't in any way lessen my worry or my fear.

'Why don't you give your mum a call?' Barry suggested. It was as if he had read my mind. 'You should let her know you're okay. She'll be worried.'

'No,' I answered, fearfully. 'Don't let them find out where I am!'

'They won't find out,' said Mrs Jones, gently. 'Not from just a phone call. Just tell them you're staying the night with a friend. Don't give them any details.'

'I'm really scared of speaking to them.'

'Of course you are,' said Barry. 'That's only natural. But you need to call them, so that they don't start looking for you. It's all part of remaining hidden.'

I was shown to the phone in Mrs Jones's hall, and with a shaking hand I dialled home.

As soon as I heard someone pick up, I blurted out: 'Hello, I'm okay, but I'm not coming home. I'm staying with friends. Bye.'

Before anyone could reply, I slammed down the phone. I didn't even know who it was I had been talking to. Barry left shortly after that, and I sat down to dinner with Mrs Jones, her husband and their son, Jonathan. I was amazed at how they went about eating their evening meal. Mrs Jones and I – the women of the household – sat around the same table as the men, eating and chatting. Her son, who was a grown man, even helped set and clear the table.

Mrs Jones served up some strange, grey liquid for dinner. It turned out to be mushroom soup. The only English food that I'd ever had was chips, and I had never tasted anything like it. It wasn't exactly my mother's spicy curry. But I didn't mind. Mrs Jones could have served me up broken glass for all I cared. I had escaped. I was safe. That was all that mattered.

I hardly said a word over dinner. Afterwards, Mrs Jones showed me to a bedroom. It was her adopted daughter, Julie's, room. There was a single bed, a wardrobe and a desk for study.

'Make yourself at home,' she said. 'Julie's away at university, and she won't mind.' She paused for a second. 'Hannan, would you like to go to college tomorrow, or do you want to stay here?'

I thought about it for a moment. 'I'd like to go to college. I'd like to do some study tomorrow, if possible.'

'That's great.' Mrs Jones gave me a hug, handed me some folded-up pyjamas, and wished me goodnight.

I'd never had pyjamas before. At home, we used to sleep in our day clothes. I'd seen them on TV, so at least I had an idea what people did with them. Mrs Jones closed the door, and at last I was on my own. I was feeling lonely, and unsure of what would happen next. There had been no conversation about how long I might stay here. Mrs Jones had said she just wanted me to get some rest, so I could get over the trauma.

But in spite of my worries, I was filled with a wonderful sense of relief. Finally, I away from the threat of abduction and forced marriage. Mrs Jones was there and I trusted her. I felt safe in her house – much safer than I had ever felt in my own home.

I had a little weep into my pillow, and drifted into a deep sleep.

Chapter Seventeen

Mrs Jones's House

The next morning breakfast was cornflakes and tea eaten at the table in the kitchen. I felt almost as if I was in a dream – sitting there eating strange food in a strange house with this family of white people.

Mrs Jones's husband was a quiet, gentle kind of man, and it struck me almost immediately how different he was from my father. He was very open about being affectionate towards his wife, and appreciative of her. Over breakfast, he commented to her what a lovely, charming girl I was. I smiled and blushed. The compliment felt natural coming from him, although no one had ever said such a thing to me before.

Mr Jones was a lecturer at Leeds University. Jonathan, their son, was in his early twenties and he worked as a builder. He was shy, gentle and quiet, like his father. But he took after his mother in appearance: he was tall and good-looking, just like her. Before leaving for work, he larked around with the dogs and made his mother laugh.

On the drive into college Mrs Jones told me the story of Julie, the girl whose room I was staying in. Julie was another teenage girl that Mrs Jones had taken in, and over time she had formally adopted her. She treated Julie as her own daughter, sending her to college and university. And before Julie, she had rescued a Chinese girl who was in trouble with her family.

I think Mrs Jones told me these stories to help reassure me. It worked. She had a golden heart, and she knew something of what she was getting into by helping me.

We drove right into the college car park, and I was able to use

the staff entrance at the back. I was terrified that I'd see my dad
and brothers gathered at the college, but thankfully there was no
sign of them. I was hugely relieved, but I knew they were going to
turn up sooner or later, and part of me wanted to get it over and
done with. Mrs Jones knew they were going to come, too. I didn't
need to warn her.

'The chances are that your family will be here today,' she told
me as she escorted me to my first lesson. 'But don't worry. We're
here for you. You have our total support.'

I went into class, and Mrs Jones went to have a word with the
principal. She explained to him that I was fleeing a forced
marriage, and that I would be staying with her for as long as I
wanted. Luckily, the principal was very understanding and supportive. It was mid-morning when he appeared at the door of my
class to have a quiet word with the teacher. I knew instinctively
that my father was there.

'Hannan, can you go to Mrs Jones's room,' said the teacher.
'The principal will take you there . . .'

When we reached Mrs Jones's office the principal explained
what had happened. 'Your father's in my office, and he's demanding to see you. I'm quite happy to send him away, if that's what
you want. It's entirely up to you.'

I glanced at Mrs Jones and back to the principal. 'Don't send
him away,' I said. 'I want to see him and get it over with. I want
him to know that I'm not going home. I want him to know that
he's never going to force me into any marriage. I want him to
hear it from me. He needs to know that it's my decision, that it's
me who's standing up to him.'

We set off for the principal's office. When we got there, the
principal opened the door, and there was my father. He was with
a man from the mosque whom he'd brought along in order to
translate. But the shock wasn't in seeing him: it was seeing my
father in tears. He was openly weeping. I had never seen him
show any emotion, other than anger, hatred or lust, yet here he
was openly crying. I couldn't believe that I had upset him that
much, and for a moment my determination wavered.

And then I just knew that those tears weren't genuine. They weren't about me. If anything, he was crying because I had brought shame on him, the family and the community. And for all I knew my father was crying for the benefit of the teachers – so that they would feel sorry for him, and see what a kind, loving father he really was. Perhaps he calculated that it might make me relent, that seeing his tears might convince me to change my mind.

'How will I hold my head up high in the community, when you have disgraced us?' my father wailed. 'Such shame! Such shame you have brought on us!'

I was beyond all that. After sixteen years of beatings and abuse, I knew how coldly manipulative my father was. And I knew how dark and dead was his heart. What said it all for me was that there wasn't the slightest hint of remorse in his eyes. In spite of the tears, he couldn't hide the cold rage that he nurtured within. But my father's biggest mistake was that he didn't for one moment say that he was sorry. Instead, he was wailing on at me in Punjabi about 'honour' and 'shame'.

'The shame, the shame!' he railed. 'Look what you've *done* to us . . . Look at the shame you've brought on the family. Please come home, Hannan, please come home. How can we live with the shame?'

At that moment I knew absolutely that my father's tears were false. It was a sickening show and a sham. He didn't care one jot about me. He cared only to maintain his precious, precious 'honour'.

'No way,' I answered him, in Punjabi. 'I'm not coming home today, and I'm not coming home tomorrow. I'm never coming home.'

I sat there for a while as Dad kept wailing on and on about the shame of what I was doing. He tried his best to work his emotional blackmail on me.

'You've brought such shame on the family! Such shame. Come home. Your mother can't stand it. She can't live with it. Please come home.'

Eventually, I turned to the principal. 'There's nothing more I want to say to him. I've told him I'm not going home. My mind's made up.'

'Well then, that's it,' said the principal. 'You can go now, if you like. And well done for coming here to speak . . .'

I left without another word to my father.

Mrs Jones came with me. 'Are you sure you're okay? You were very brave in there.'

'I'm fine,' I told her. 'I'm glad it's over. Can I go back to class now?'

Of course, that wasn't the end of it. Over the next few days my father sent every imaginable family member and relative to the college. First there were my brothers, one by one. Another day, it was Mum with my sisters. Then there were my uncles. I refused to see any of them. I left instructions with the college reception that I didn't want to see my family, or my relatives. I cut off all communication.

I was too busy trying to get used to not living at home, and adjusting to my new family and my new life. I didn't have time to worry about the effect my running away might be having on my father or the wider community. And anyway, why should I care?

Whenever I did pause to think about it, I didn't relish the fact that they would be burning in shame. I didn't want to hurt my family, or cause them embarrassment. I didn't want them to suffer. But at the same time I didn't feel guilty for what I had done. It was the right thing, of that I was absolutely certain. Mostly, it was about me getting away from the abuse. The catalyst for my running away had been the forced marriage, but the problems were far deeper and darker than that alone.

It was a Tuesday when I had run away. On the Saturday, Mrs Jones took the family to a café, for lunch, and she asked me to go with them. I'd never done anything like this before. I'd never once eaten out, with or without my family. It felt so odd going somewhere to have someone you'd never met cook you a meal, and paying what seemed like a fortune for the privilege. I found myself watching what the others were doing, and trying to do as they did. That's how I got through my first ever meal in a restaurant.

The Jones family chatted away, and lingered over their food. They told me to call them by their first names – James, Felicity, and Jonathan, or Johnny for short. James talked about his week at work, and the goings-on at their church. Both he and Felicity were Christians. Felicity talked about Johnny's girlfriend, Zoë, and having her over for Sunday lunch. Friends of theirs came in and out of the restaurant, and they paused to chat. It was all so different from what I knew.

Of course, they were simply behaving like any English family might. I found myself enjoying the ebb and flow of the conversation. At home we rarely if ever sat down as a family and chatted. Mostly, Mum and Dad ordered us around. And as for mealtimes, Dad rarely if ever ate with the women – he'd be served his food in 'his' room. And the rest of us usually ate in front of the TV.

In fact, Dad had a rule that meals were for eating, not talking. According to him, talking while eating was haram. So we used to eat in silence. My brothers might talk to each other, whilst watching the TV. But if Dad was there, more than likely there would be no conversation at all. No one was relaxed when he was around.

In my new life I had so much freedom from the very start. I almost didn't know what to do with it. In the suburbs where the Joneses lived no one knew me. I could wander around at will, quite unnoticed. I was suddenly free of all the slave-like chores that I had been forced to do at home. I could still help out, of course, but I wasn't forced to, and I wasn't beaten if I made a mistake. Freedom, choice and anonymity were new things that I would have to learn to cope with.

Mrs Jones encouraged me to stay in touch with my family. I called up one evening and my brother Raz answered the phone.

'Hi Raz, it's Hannan,' I said. 'I'm okay. I just want you all to know I'm okay. I'm staying with friends.'

'Where are you?' Raz asked. He sounded worried, not angry. 'Why won't you come home?'

'I'm at a friend's house, Raz. And I'm not coming home. I'm staying where I am.'

'Talk to Mum, will you?' Raz suggested. 'She's right here.'

'No. I'm going now, Raz. Bye.'

I put the phone down. I didn't want to talk to Mum. I knew how she'd guilt-trip me – using tears and emotional blackmail. I knew she'd do all she could to try to get me back. *I'm so ill and it's your fault. I'm sick with worry. I miss you so much. Come home.* It would be hard to hear. And I didn't need it right now.

The one real link to my old life was Skip, my fellow runaway rebel. I spoke to her on the phone quite a lot. She'd keep me up to date with what was going on in the street, although I wasn't particularly interested.

'Your parents keep asking me if I know where you are,' she'd tell me. 'It's a good thing I don't. Let's keep it that way. Then I won't need to lie!'

I wasn't surprised that they were trying to track me down. It was what I had expected. But my parents didn't know the Joneses' side of town at all. No Asians lived here, so they had no contacts who might report on me. It did cross my mind that all they really had to do was wait outside the college gates and follow Felicity's car. She was driving us to college and back each day. So we started to keep an eye open for any cars following us, in particular a purple Skoda! But there didn't seem to be any.

A few weeks after my escape Felicity took me shopping, to get me some clothes. I had next to nothing to wear and had been borrowing Julie's clothes. I had never been clothes shopping before. I had only ever been to a material shop, to buy cloth for the canary yellow shalwar kamiz that Mum made me wear. Felicity began showing me tops and jumpers and jeans, and asking me which ones I liked. I didn't really know what to say. I was too embarrassed having her buy these things for me.

'You need some warm clothes,' Felicity told me, picking out a thick cotton nightie decorated with fluffy sheep.

She was right. It was the end of November and freezing. On the way home Felicity chatted away about Johnny and Zoë. They had been going out for several years, and Felicity was hoping that they would soon get married. So this was what it was like being free to choose your life partner. It was all so different from what I was used to, and from the abduction and forced marriage I had so narrowly escaped.

'I'm never, ever going to get married,' I remarked quietly.

I meant it, too. After what my father had done to me, the thought of having a physical relationship with any man was just repulsive. I didn't think I could ever trust a man in that way. All I had ever known was dirt and pain and abuse and darkness. I hadn't told Felicity about my father abusing me. I guessed she presumed that my anti-marriage sentiment was due to a narrow escape from a forced marriage.

Felicity laughed. 'You might change your mind in the future!'

'I wouldn't bet on it,' I replied.

'Well, you never know. One day you might meet the man of your dreams and fall in love.'

Chapter Eighteen

Apostasy Pending

One Sunday shortly after I had run away, Felicity took the family to church.

'Make yourself at home, Hannan,' she said. 'We won't be long.'

On the spur of the moment I asked if I could go. It wasn't that I was frightened of being on my own. In fact, I was happy with my own company and in my own little world. I asked more out of curiosity. I wanted to see if her church was the same as the one I had been to at primary school, with lots of incomprehensible prayers in Latin. Going to that church had been as dull as going to hear a Quran reading. The only difference was that you didn't get beaten if you fell asleep.

Felicity hesitated. 'You really don't have to come, you know. It's not necessary.'

'But I want to go. I want to see what it's like.'

Felicity took some convincing. Because she was my Religious Studies teacher, she was being doubly careful about not influencing me in any way. She wanted me to make my own choice about whether I went or not, and she made me convince her that I really was going of my own free will.

Part of the reason I wanted to go was curiosity. Here was this person who'd let me stay in her house, in spite of the potential risks. I wanted to know more about her, her family, and their belief system. The very idea of my parents inviting a stranger of another race and faith to share their home with them was a total impossibility. I wondered what gave Mrs Jones such an incredible generosity of spirit.

All my life my parents had told me that I was a useless, godless child destined to end up in Hell. I believed it at the time. I believed that I would never be good enough for their god. When Felicity had told me that God loved me, all those months ago at college, I had reacted with shock. How could there be a *loving* god? It didn't seem possible. My parents' god was one of punishment and damnation – a god I could never be good enough for. I was intrigued by Felicity's idea of God, even whilst I didn't believe it could be true.

The church was an ancient building carved out of immutable grey stone. It was a Methodist church, so Felicity told me, although I didn't really understand what that meant. We went up some steps to the chapel, where there were rows of wooden pews. The church was packed, and there was hardly room to get me in.

I found space on a pew next to Felicity, and glanced around me. There were no other Asians present, only whites. At first I did feel rather strange, and I did get some odd looks. But once Felicity had introduced me everyone was very friendly. Mostly, I was happy not to speak or be spoken to. I was filled with a quiet curiosity.

Felicity's husband was playing a piano at the front of the church. As the music flowed and swelled, I gazed at the beautiful stained-glass windows, and the ornate carved pillars. I thought what a grand place this church was. It struck me that it had a special presence. A hymn was sung. I listened, but I didn't know any of the words. Felicity tried to point them out to me, running her finger along the lines in the hymn book as she sang. Then there was a reading from the Bible, followed by the sermon.

The priest was called Bob. He was in his mid-fifties, and I was immediately struck by how human and intimate his sermon seemed. He started off by telling a story about something quite ridiculous that had happened to him over the weekend. Suddenly, everyone was laughing as he regaled the congregation with his mishaps. I was amazed. It was inconceivable to laugh at a Muslim holy man – like my father. And it would be inconceivable for him to tell such an entertaining, self-deprecating, human story.

Bob used the story as the basis for his sermon. People seemed alive to his message, and there was real laughter and joy at his words. As Bob continued talking, there was excitement in his voice, and a real love in what he was telling people. When it came to the singing, Bob stood out front and played his guitar. The only trouble was he only knew a few chords, and so he'd have to stop every now and then and do 'air guitar'. He even made fun of himself for doing so.

For me it was unthinkable for an Imam in his mid-fifties to behave like Bob. All those that I had met took themselves, and their words, far too seriously. After the hymns there were prayers, followed by church notices, and one final hymn. It was Amazing Grace. As the congregation sang, the words came floating back to me, for I had sung Amazing Grace with my junior school choir. Most of the congregation seemed to have that song off by heart. By the volume of the singing, it seemed to be a church favourite.

I left that church service feeling somehow happy and intrigued. I was fascinated to know how Bob the priest could be so easy and relaxed, even to the extent of making fun of himself in a house of God, and in front of his congregation. Bob seemed so excited by his faith, and by the life of Jesus in particular. I had once been told by my father that I wasn't even allowed to mention Jesus' name in our house. So what was it that made him so exciting in Bob the preacher's eyes?

The following Saturday I asked Felicity if I could go with her again to church. She seemed happy to take me. It was the same format, but with a different sermon from Bob, and Amazing Grace to finish. Bob told more funny stories about himself, and he talked about Jesus and got really excited all over again. No doubt about it, Bob was a live wire. Oddly, I found myself enjoying being at Bob's church. I had never actually *liked* being in a place of worship before.

I was still a Muslim, and I just presumed I would remain a Muslim all my life. But I didn't feel like I was doing anything wrong going to a church. I'd been taken to churches on junior school outings, so it wasn't completely alien to me. Lots of things surprised me though. I saw people putting their Bibles on the floor. I found this really shocking. In my mind they were disrespecting a holy book. We would never dream of putting a Quran on the floor.

The lessons and readings were all in English, and I could actually understand everything. The prayers made especial sense to me. People prayed for those who were ill, and even for people from other countries and religions who were poor or unfortunate. They prayed for whatever misfortune had happened that week – an earthquake in South America, or flooding in Bangladesh. There seemed to be a concern for the wider world, disregarding whether it was Christian or otherwise.

I'd never heard anything even remotely like this in a Muslim setting. The prayers at the mosque would be set verses from the Quran. You would always repeat the same ones. It never seemed to vary.

God is great,
God is great,
There is only one God . . .

But I was most surprised at the concept of Christians praying for people of other faiths. It seemed very odd to me. Within my own experience of Islam that never happened. There is a concept of *zakat* – charity – in Islam, but from my experience it was always to help other Muslims. In fact, in the Quran charity is supposed to be extended to anyone who is poor and needy, but for me it had never been like that in practice.

And it certainly wasn't the way it was taught by my father. According to him, zakat was an exclusively Muslim thing. Charity was only ever extended to the *ummah* – the global community under Islam. At the mosque they would raise money for earthquakes and other disasters, but it would have to be for a Muslim country. An earthquake in Peru, for instance, wouldn't merit the slightest interest, or support.

I stayed with Mrs Jones for several months, and those were some of the happiest days of my life. I even went on holiday with them. We spent two weeks by the seaside in Cornwall, camping at a place called Coverack, near Lands End. It was the first time I had really seen the sea. I actually went swimming, or at least paddling, in the waves.

But camping was a challenge for me. I didn't mind sleeping out in a field, and I liked being close to nature. But after the years of abuse I had developed a horrible claustrophobia. It hit me hard that first night. I was in a one-man tent on my own, and I hardly slept at all.

The next morning I told Felicity that I hadn't been able to sleep. She was very understanding, and from then on I went in with Zoë, sharing a much bigger tent. It had two sleeping pods, one at either end, and a living area in the middle. I left the zip undone in my pod, so I felt as if I could escape if I needed to. I was just about able to cope with that.

The campsite had a breathtaking view over the sea. Each morning we'd eat outside, gazing out over the vast, powerful expanse of ocean rolling out before us. It took my breath away. I found it beautiful and free, as opposed to daunting. Breakfast was always a fry-up cooked over a gas stove. As a Muslim, I couldn't eat bacon or sausages, but I had to admit that the smell of them frying was mouth-watering.

After a morning on the beach we might go to the local art gallery, situated not far from the campsite. It was located in a beautiful stone cottage and it had a teashop attached. We would wander around the gallery admiring the seascapes and other works, and have an enormous cream tea to follow.

It was so relaxing and so serene camped out on those cliff-tops in the fresh sea breeze. I felt as if I was in a kind of paradise. I didn't think much about my old life. I was just so relieved to be out of it. All I wanted to do was to forget about it and push it away. The slavery, the threats, the fear and isolation, and the abuse – all of that I wanted to leave behind me as I embraced my new world.

By now I was getting to know Zoë well, and we were becoming close. It was a kind of friendship I'd never known before. I felt as if I could trust her with anything. I was tempted to tell her the whole truth about my life of abuse in my father's house, but I wasn't ready yet. I wanted to live my happy new life for a while at least, before going back into the darkness.

For the first time, I felt truly free. I didn't want my father's dark shadow cast over me again, even if it was just the memories.

Whenever I was at the Joneses' home on a Sunday and they set off to church I would go with them. Week after week, I sat quietly in my pew and watched and listened. The care and the love that I experienced in the Jones family, and at their church, had to come from somewhere, I reasoned. If it came from their God, then perhaps I should try to get to know him. I started attending the church youth group, where I met a girl called Rachel.

Rachel was from a typical white northern English family. Her dad was a social worker, and a real gentleman. Her mum was a teaching assistant in a primary school. Rachel was a petite, blonde bombshell. She was two years younger than me, and she was very popular at school – with both the girls and the boys!

I found it funny that this petite blonde angel spoke with such a strong northern accent. Mine was still tinged with a Pakistani lilt, but the longer I spent away from my street the more that was fading. I was happy to hear it go. Apart from my skin colour – which I could never change, nor would I ever want to – I was happy to dispense with just about anything that reminded me of my former life.

Rachel helped ease me into the process of being a free young woman. She took me clothes shopping, and helped me experiment with makeup and jewellery. We played board games at her house. Scrabble was my favourite. I found that I had a wide vocabulary – it must have been all those lonely hours spent reading. Sometimes, I would sleep over at Rachel's house. We'd talk and talk for hours on end. Quite often her mum was there, and she'd be chatting with us almost as if we were all good friends.

Whenever we could afford it, Rachel and I would go to the cinema. I had never once been to the movies, and I was stunned by Titanic, one of the first films we saw. The special effects were a big deal at the time, and it was so amazing to see it on the big screen. But what appealed to me most was the romance – the idea that Leonardo DiCaprio's character could die to save his love. I really liked his sense of humour, too. And the fact he was an artist. When he drew a picture of his love, played by Kate Winslet, it really touched me. It was the kind of love that I wanted to find – maybe one day.

At around this time Felicity suggested I should go to the social services, to apply for educational grants and housing benefit. I was studying and living with no means of financial support, apart from her generosity. Felicity dropped me off at the benefits office. I told the benefits supervisor, a young white man, the full story of my having fled home and a forced marriage. He took me into an inside office, where he started to fire questions at me. Finally, he started demanding my family's details.

'You have to give me your parents' phone number,' he said. 'I can't process anything without that.'

'But what do you need it for?' I asked.

'Well, if nothing else I have to verify your story. I can't just take it at face value, can I?'

'But you don't understand,' I protested. 'I just told you I've run away from an arranged marriage. I can't risk them knowing where I am, or what I'm doing.'

He shrugged. 'We can't give you benefits without verification. It's very unlikely we can help you, anyway. Most likely you'll have to go home to live with your parents.'

I was getting really scared now. What on earth was this idiot going on about? What made it all the worse was that he kept going in and out to speak to someone else, then coming back with more questions. Finally he told me point blank that I had to go back to my father's house. My family should be supporting me, not the benefits office. He kept demanding the phone number, so he could call them up and 'arrange things'.

'There's no way I'm giving you my parents' number,' I said. 'It's getting late. I have to go.'

With that I got up and scurried out of the office. Just as soon as I was outside I burst into tears. I went to the nearest phone box, and called Felicity.

'Wait right there!' she ordered, once I'd told her what had happened. I could tell how angry she was. 'I'm coming right over to have words with them.'

She drove straight from college, and we went back in together.

'Don't worry, no one's sending you home,' she reassured me. 'I won't let them.'

Felicity asked me which man I had spoken to. I pointed him out behind one of the counters. She marched straight up to him. It was the end of the day, so fortunately there weren't too many people around.

'How dare you tell this young girl she has to go home,' she announced. 'You know nothing about her situation. You don't have a clue – and yet you're telling her she has to go home!'

'And who are you?' the man demanded, rudely.

'I'm her college tutor,' Felicity fired back at him. 'And I'm also her guardian. If you persist with this behaviour, I will immediately inform the college principal, and her social worker. This is totally unacceptable. We may even have to report it to the police. This girl's very life could have been endangered by your actions.'

The man was looking worried now. He could tell that Felicity meant business. 'Look, I'm sorry,' he said. 'I didn't fully appreciate her situation. I was just trying to verify some details, and check she wasn't lying to me about her story . . .'

'Verifying she's telling the truth doesn't require forcing her to return to a dangerous and abusive family, does it?' Felicity countered, icily. 'Or am I missing something?'

'Erm . . . Look, why don't we start over?' said the man, nervously. 'We'll fill in a whole new set of forms, and get the application under way for educational grants and housing benefit. Let's just forget I ever said anything about her family, okay?'

By the time we left the office, I was exhausted. But at least it was done. Now there'd be a little money coming in from the council to support me.

I learned many things during those months that I lived with Mrs Jones. I learned that not all white English people spent their lives getting drunk and sleeping around. This is what my father had told me, but like so much else it was blind prejudice and lies. There was another England, different from the one depicted by my father. It was an England populated by the Mrs Joneses of this world – good, honest, open-minded, tolerant people, whose faith lifted them up and gave their lives meaning.

I thanked God for Mrs Jones. But I wasn't exactly sure whose God it was that I was thanking.

Chapter Nineteen

This is My Church

I spent Christmas with my 'adopted' family – the Joneses.

In my home and on my street Christmas had been no different from any other holiday – except that there were better films on TV. We were a Muslim family in a Muslim community, and there was no Christmas tree at home, no decorations, and no presents. There was nothing to acknowledge the event that was being celebrated all across the country.

I did get the odd Christmas card from school friends. And Mum would secretly give me some money with which to buy cards and stamps, so I could send some of my own. But I wasn't allowed to put those cards up at home. Instead, I hid them in my school bag and pushed it under the bed. Once Christmas was over, I threw them in the rubbish so that Dad wouldn't find them.

Presents had never been a part of our life, either. For the Muslim festival of Eid, we would usually get given a little money. On birthdays, I might get something from my schoolmates – a card or a present – but birthdays were never acknowledged at home. Some people on our street did celebrate their children's birthdays, but generally they weren't a big deal in our culture.

In Felicity's home I saw the Christmas tree going up, along with decorations all over the house. We wrapped up presents and heaped them up beneath the tree. I helped Rachel put her tree up, too. I really enjoyed it. There was an electric buzz of anticipation in the air. I'd never felt anything like this at home. It was so cold outside, and coming into a festive house to sit in front of an open fire felt lovely. It was just so perfect.

I bought the Jones family a box of chocolates for Christmas – which was all I could afford. I knew Rachel had got me something, so I got her some earrings. On Christmas Eve we went to church for midnight mass. I listened to Bob telling the story of Jesus' birth. As he spoke it seemed to me that he believed so passionately in what he was saying, and in the love of his caring God. I had seen the nativity plays at primary school, but all it had been was the story of the birth of this holy man called Jesus.

As I listened to the story as related by Bob, I really heard it. Quite a few times he repeated the phrase: 'God became man'. That idea filled my mind. I was amazed that God could become something as humble as a normal man. As Bob was such a humble person, likewise was his God. Bob's God had brought himself down to the level of a humble man, so he could better bring his words to earth. That really touched me. It was so different from what I had heard in my father's ranting and raving.

Bob kept talking about love: the love of a God that made him want to come to earth as a man, to communicate with us and to care for us. He stressed this word over and over in his sermon. Love. Love. *God's love.* Felicity's adopted daughter, Julie, was sitting next to me on the pew. Eventually, I leant across and whispered in her ear.

'How does someone *become* a Christian?'

Julie smiled. 'Easy. You just ask Jesus to come into your life. Ask him to forgive your wrongs, and give thanks that he died on the cross and rose again for you.'

'And that's it?'

Julie nodded. 'That's it.'

'There's no set words you have to say, no witnesses, or anything?'

'No. None. You can get baptised if you like, but you don't *have* to.'

This seemed to me to be such a private, personal thing, and I rather liked it being so. In order to become a Muslim, one has to repeat the following phrase three times, ideally in front of a Muslim witness: 'I bear witness that there is no God but God, and that Mohammed is his true prophet.' Once that was done, you would go before an Imam and be declared a Muslim. I had presumed there would be a similar formality to Christianity, but it seemed there was none.

I returned to the Jones house, and went to bed dreaming of the piles of presents under the tree! But I couldn't sleep. I kept thinking about Bob's words, and what Julie had said to me. So I prayed, and, for the first time in my life, I prayed to a Christian God: 'God, if you are real, if you exist and you are a loving God, then I want to know you, and I want you to come into my heart.'

And that I guess was the moment when I converted. I didn't really think about it like that at the time. It was just an instinctive act in the moment. I didn't think about the past – the last sixteen years of being a Muslim. I didn't think about the faith of my birth. I was just lost in the emotion of the moment. I didn't even consider what my changing faith might mean. I was carried along in an unstoppable flow that propelled me to a new place – a place of love and laughter and light.

For the next few days I didn't really think much about what I had done. There were presents to open and visitors and Christmas lunches, all of which kept me busy. I left to one side contemplating the massive change this signified in my life, and the impact it might have on my relationships, most of all with my family. I was just caught up in the spirit of my first Christmas. I didn't breathe a word to anyone about the change that had been wrought within me – not even to Mrs Jones.

On Christmas Day we exchanged our presents. I had never unwrapped a present before, so I watched what the others did. I saw them opening their parcels in front of each other, and smiling and saying thank you. I tried to follow suit, but I felt odd and awkward. I didn't know how to respond to a family member giving me anything, except punishment or abuse. I didn't know what to do or how to act. All I did know is that I was happy. Happier than I'd ever thought I could be.

I started to read the Bible, and I just found that it spoke to me. At this point, I wasn't really comparing it to the Quran. I was just learning about what it meant to be a Christian, about how Jesus would want me to live my life. I was embracing this newfound freedom to be myself, and most of all the right to be loved. It wasn't about being worthy or deserving any more. It wasn't about being rejected. It was about knowing the love of God was there in spite of everything. More than anything, I felt an inner peace.

For the first time in my life, I truly felt at peace with myself.

There was nothing public about my conversion: no announcement and no ceremony. It was a completely private thing. Two weeks after Christmas, I was having lunch with the family, and I decided to say something to Felicity. I felt ready to tell someone, and she was the person who, more than anyone, I wanted to know. James and Jonathan were there, too.

I glanced around the table a little nervously. 'On Christmas Eve . . . Well, erm, I – I think I became a Christian.'

There was no reason for me to be nervous, of course. A huge smile broke out on Felicity's face, and she jumped up and hugged me. We danced and danced around her living room, and then I had to be hugged by each of the members of the family in turn. Close physical contact was shunned in my family, unless it was Dad's abusive hands upon me. I liked this hugging thing, but I was still a little uncomfortable with it.

One part of me thought the Jones family were a bit crazy, the way they were dancing and laughing so excitedly. But the other part of me liked the uninhibited way in which they showed their emotions. There was a freedom and a lightness in it that I found refreshing. Some families on my street had been a bit like this. Amina and Ruhama's father would hug them and show affection openly. It was only really in my father's house, and under his regime, that such things were forbidden.

Dad just didn't do emotion, or closeness – not with anyone. The main feeling he projected into the family was anger. He was a very, very angry man. In truth, he had to be angry at himself.

Deep down, he must have known he was an evil fraud. But he projected that anger onto those whom he defined as doing wrong: other cultures, other races, other religions and ways, or his family when they broke the 'rules'. In the wider community that anger went largely unseen, for then he wore his gentle, smiley skin.

Felicity didn't say it openly, but she knew what a momentous change my conversion represented. She knew it could cause me real trouble, and this worried her greatly. I had run away from my family, my culture, and the merry-go-round of honour and shame. Now, I had run from my religion, too. She knew it wasn't going to be easy. But for now she was happy to concentrate on being overjoyed for me.

I'm glad she didn't voice her concerns then. She gave me the freedom and support I needed to make my own way, to make my own religious choice, to follow my own free will – and to make my own mistakes if necessary. I had been rigidly controlled and punished for so long. Now, at last, I had the freedom to discover who and what I wanted to be. I was learning to become my own person.

Even after telling the Jones family, my conversion remained largely a private thing. But a few weeks later I decided to tell some of my college friends. A number of them were Muslims, but none of them seemed to react particularly strongly at the time. Over the weeks that followed, however, one by one my Muslim friends stopped talking to me, and stopped sitting next to me in class.

I had half expected this. I wasn't that surprised. In a way, I had chosen to tell them to confirm what I knew was going to happen – that once my conversion was known about, the Muslim community would ostracise me. If that was the case, then those friendships weren't genuine, and never had been. They were conditional on a set of factors – religion, honour and shame. They were friendships that I didn't particularly want any more, or value.

With Felicity, Julie, Rachel and Zoë, I had seen people extend friendship and offer me sanctuary in the face of great danger and risk – regardless of the fact that I was from a different race, religion and culture. That was the meaning of true friendship – one that I decided to embrace.

In my eyes, it was so much more real.

Chapter Twenty

Moving On, Breaking Up

Several months later I moved on from Felicity's house. I took a room I had been offered by the Project for Accommodation in Bermford (PAB), a housing association for young people bereft of family support. I was placed with a married couple who were supposed to care for me as part of their family. They received housing benefit and family support for doing so.

I had loved living in Felicity's house and feeling a part of her family, but all good things come to an end. I wanted to experiment with my life and to really push the boundaries of my independence and freedom. I wanted to stand on my own two feet more than ever, and to do so I felt that I had – reluctantly – to leave Felicity's home.

I wanted to learn to manage my own finances, to cook and care for myself, to become totally self-sufficient, and to be able to manage my own freedom. That's what most people my age could do, and I wanted the same. I wanted to be like them. PAB put you with people who could help you learn all those 'life skills' and make the transition into a free and independent person.

I stayed in my new, PAB accommodation for eighteen months, during which time I increasingly focused on my college studies. At first, I was finishing off my GCSE re-sits. I planned to go on to do A-levels at the college, and I knew that I absolutely had to do well. I had turned my back on my family, my religion and an arranged marriage. I had given up everything I knew from the old life, and now I would have to survive on my wits alone.

I still had lots of contact with Felicity and her family. Johnny would pick me up from my new home to take me to church.

And three or four times a week I travelled back from college with Felicity, and ate dinner at her house. Even so, I began to worry that perhaps my bid for total freedom had been premature. Too much had happened to me over too short a period of time, and it all started to pile up on me. What was more, I was denying the real horror that I had been through – the abuse – in an effort to embrace a happy, bright and free future.

Not long after I had left Felicity's house my problems began. I felt as if I had had my support network pulled out from under me, although it was me who had done all the pulling. I suppose it was hardly surprising when things started to fall apart. Over time I became depressed, so much so that I couldn't even talk to people about how dark and dirty I felt inside.

That January I volunteered to enter a mental health ward. I wasn't sectioned: it was by choice. But every time the staff mentioned telling my family that I was there, I'd start to scream and scream. The hospital assigned me a psychiatrist. Yet all I was willing to tell him was that I had been sexually abused as a child, and that I wasn't ready to talk about it. I didn't even reveal who it was who had abused me.

I was also feeling confused. Who was I, I wondered. I was anAsian born a Muslim who had converted to Christianity, and whose every friend was white. Where on earth did I belong? My friends at church loved me and cared for me, but they had not the slightest understanding of my background. Meanwhile, my family rejected the person I had become, and would do even more if they discovered I had converted out of Islam.

I didn't regret leaving home, or becoming a Christian. Far from it. But this was still a test for me. I took great comfort in the story of Jesus' persecuted life – how he was rejected, betrayed by those closest to him and crucified, yet how he endured it all.

I was diagnosed with clinical depression, and put on anti-depressants. They made me so tired. I seemed to sleep the whole time. Felicity came nearly every day to see me, and Zoë, Johnny and Rachel often came with her. My tutors and the college principal also came to visit, as did the wife of the couple I had been living with. And even Barry, my social worker, paid a visit.

For some reason I had an obsession with Penguin snack bars – so everyone would bring me packets of those to eat. That's what I seemed to live on. These kind people were the rocks around which I tried to tether my confused and darkened mind. I knew they would be there to support me whatever happened, and that was what gave me the courage to get better.

But the mental ward was a very strange place to be. I made friends with a schizophrenic guy. When he was on his medication he was great, but off it he was a monster. One night he forgot to take his pills, and he came over and punched me on the nose.

On another occasion I was reading my Bible in the day room, and a guy who was coming off heroin came to sit beside me. He was a giant, tattooed skinhead, and his outward appearance was terrifying. I was reminded of the men who had beaten up my brother Zakir, whilst hurling 'Paki Saddam-lover' abuse at us.

'I'm Freddie,' he announced.

He began to talk to me about his life. When he had finished, he asked me what I was reading. He asked if he could borrow my Bible, and the next day he came and asked me how he could become a Christian. I repeated what Julie had told me all those months ago in church, and left the rest up to Freddie.

I struck up an incredible friendship with him. But Freddie was the type of person that my parents would have condemned as being a druggy, infidel 'low-life'. In fact, he was a lovely, gentle giant of a person, and he and I supported each other during the toughest times. Freddie went on to get married and have children, and then he became a vicar. What a turn-around for a life that had once seemed so hopeless.

With time, my spirits seemed to heal. After several weeks I decided that I was ready to leave. I checked out of the hospital and tried to get on with my life. I felt like I had just started a long journey towards telling the full truth of what had happened to me. In a very limited way I had spoken out about it to the hospital psychiatrist, so at least I had taken the first step. I was on the path now. I just needed the strength to continue.

I built up my spirits gradually. I spent a lot of time at Felicity's house, and I was very grateful for her support. One morning we were sitting around having breakfast. Felicity had been frying bacon for the rest of the family. She placed the constituent parts for making bacon sandwiches – white or brown bread, fried rashers and tomato sauce – on the table. Everyone tucked in, and as always it smelled so good.

Without really thinking I reached out and made myself a bacon sandwich: a slice of bread; butter slapped on; a rasher on top; a splurge of tomato sauce, and a slice to cap it all. Just as soon as I bit into that bacon sandwich I realised what I had been missing all these years. It was one of the most delicious things I'd ever tasted. There was nothing like it.

I glanced around, waiting for someone to say something; but no one said a word. I'm sure they noticed me eating that bacon sandwich. Maybe they were just being polite, or maybe they thought it would put me off enjoying it if they commented. In fact, very little could have put me off that bacon sandwich. It was divine.

I didn't really consider the significance of what I was doing while I was eating it. But later I thought to myself: *oh my goodness, I've eaten pork!* For a few hours I fully expected to be sick. I was sure something horrid would happen. But nothing did. After a while I wondered what all the fuss was about. After that, I was a top fan of bacon butties.

The other taboo that it took me ages to get over was showing my legs. It would be almost two years before I finally wore a skirt out and about in public.

A few months after getting out of the psychiatric hospital I decided to try to make direct contact with my family again. I had phoned Mum a couple of times from the hospital, but I never gave her my number. All she ever talked about was when I was going to come home.

'You're making me so ill like this, you know,' she'd complain.

'My health's suffering. We all miss you so much. When are you going to come home?'

I'd tell her what I'd told her each and every time before. 'Mum, I'm not coming home. You know why I'm not coming home. *You know*. You have to come to terms with it. I do want to stay in touch. But I'm not coming home.'

Mum's behaviour was the same old emotional blackmail. She never once said anything that suggested she cared for me, or that she was sorry. What she did say upset me, because it seemed so little had changed in her mindset. I was moving on, but my mother was still blaming me for all her ills. I was still the guilty one. The wrongdoer. And I was pretty certain that if I did go home I would pretty quickly revert to being the evil one who was unfit for their God.

One day after college I met up with Skip. By now she had got her own place, which she shared with her sister. At Skip's suggestion we went out to O'Reilly's, an Irish bar.

'What are we doing here?' I asked. It was my first ever time in a pub.

'Relax, it's fine,' said Skip. 'It's the best place to come. At least we won't run into any Muslims here!'

Skip ordered herself a pint of lager. 'Try it, and see what you think!'

I had a sip. 'Ugh! It's vile! Why would anyone want to drink that?'

Skip laughed. 'Well, I really like it – so that's what I'm having. What about you?'

I had an orange juice. There was no way that I was going to get to like lager, that much was clear.

I had started hanging out with Skip again quite a lot. She was my one surviving link to home, although she was no longer strongly tied to the community, either. Skip abhorred the authoritarian, totalitarian, misogynistic nature of the version of Islam that she and I had experienced in our community. But still she was exploring the spiritual side of her nature, and was particularly drawn to Hinduism and Buddhism.

Skip's apartment had become a haven for girls from our community who had been forced into abusive marriages, or threatened with them. One time I visited and there were three sisters there who were in a terrible situation. They were older than me, and all were well into their arranged marriages. I soon found out the bitter truth of what this had meant for them.

Each had been sent to Pakistan to marry a man they had never met before. In each case it was a distant relative from a remote village. They had then returned to the UK with their husbands. Five, six and seven years later and their marriages were sheer hell. The three sisters lived together in one house with their husbands, because they couldn't afford to buy their own place.

In my home town there was still a need for manual labour in factories. The workers didn't need to speak any English, but it was badly paid work. Still, it was all the three husbands were fit for, with no education and no English. Each of the sisters had completed secretarial studies, and they were infinitely more employable than their men. They had worked before marriage, but there was no way their husbands would allow them to do so now. And that was the poverty trap they were in.

As their story unfolded it just got worse and worse. Their very lives were being destroyed. Of course, they were regularly beaten by their husbands. They were treated as domestic slaves, waiting on them hand and foot and answering to their every need. They were hit for the slightest 'mistake', or just when their men felt like it. Worse still, their husbands were boozing on cheap alcohol. And when they were drunk, the husbands tried to share the sisters around in bed.

The sisters were disgusted and terrified. They refused to be treated like whores. They bolted the bedroom doors so that the men couldn't come in, which just made them all the more violent. Sometimes, the sisters would all sleep in the same bed for safety. They would keep knifes under the pillow, just in case they had to defend themselves. But their fear was that they wouldn't be able to fight their men off for ever. In their situation, husbands were all-powerful. They couldn't tell their parents what was happening, for it would bring 'shame' on the family to reveal such marital problems. And anyway, they felt deeply ashamed about it themselves.

They knew that sex without consent was rape, and they knew that rape was illegal in the UK. But they felt they couldn't go to the police, for nothing would bring more shame on the community than that. And they could hardly go to the Imam – *my father*. If he did anything, he would bring the matter before the mosque leaders – which would mean that the sisters had brought unspeakable 'shame' on their family by making it public. There was no one they could appeal to without bringing the whole of their lives crashing down around their ears.

Skip was horrified. I was horrified. We realised how lucky we had been to escape our own forced marriages. But what advice could we give them? All we could say was that they should leave their husbands. But they were too afraid to do so: afraid of the shame, the dishonour, the rejection by their families, and of being ostracised by the community.

I knew that the sisters wouldn't do anything to get out of their situation. They couldn't bring themselves to risk their lives and the honour of their community. Seeing how frightened they were, how miserable, and how trapped, I was doubly relieved to have made my own escape. It had placed a different set of challenges before me, but they were infinitely more preferable and benign.

I decided that I wanted to tell my family that I'd become a Christian. I felt it was important for me to make them understand how far I had moved away from them. I needed them to know that there was no route back, and that their hopes that I'd just had a temporary flip-out were absolutely in vain. I would never come back to them. I would never again play the dutiful daughter. I would never agree to marry my distant cousin, so as to shield my family from 'shame'.

My family had attempted to incarcerate me in the coffin of shame and honour. My conversion out of Islam was the final demonstration of my refusal to be so imprisoned. I called Billy and arranged to meet him in a local park. He greeted me with a big smile. I asked him how everyone was.

He shrugged. 'You know, same old same old ... Mum's asthma is getting worse. Everyone blames it on you. Ever thought about coming home?'

'I don't want to, Billy. I'm never going to do that. But there's something important I want to tell you. I've become a Christian.'

He laughed. 'Come on – you can't be serious!'

'I am serious. I've converted.'

'It's all part of your rebellion,' Billy countered. 'I know you're going through a bad patch, but you'll see sense and come home. You're a Muslim. Hannan. A Muslim.'

'Billy. You're not listening. I've converted to Christianity. I am a Christian. D'you really think I'd be welcome home now?'

Billy shook his head in despair. 'You were born a Muslim, Hannan. You'll always be one. You'll die one, too. This conversion stuff – it's bullshit.'

'I am a Christian, Billy. I've made my choice. And sooner or later you'll have to accept it.'

Billy wasn't angry or aggressive. He just thought it was another chapter in the story of the rebellion of his young sister. I'd grow out of it. With time, he thought, it would pass. We parted, saying that we'd stay in touch.

Initially, I was upset that Billy hadn't taken me seriously. But at least I'd told him. I'd communicated the message. That was what I'd wanted. It was time to get on with things.

I had so much to do in my life now.

Chapter Twenty-one

Baptism of Blood

A rough hand seized me and shoved me towards a small wooden door. It looked horribly familiar somehow. I tried to scream, but no sound came out of my mouth. The hand grabbed my hair and jerked my head backwards. I could see the fury and the contempt in the eyes. I was dragged down the rough brick steps, down into the cold shadows. Dirt and darkness overwhelmed me. I was back in the hands of my abuser.

With a jolt, I woke up. I was having recurring nightmares. The story was always the same: a flashback to the horrors of being abused in the suffocating dark of the cellar. Isolated in my suffering, I was feeling more and more desperate and increasingly alone.

I had never spoken to anyone about the sexual side of Dad's abuse. I had told the two social workers, Omer and Barry, that Dad had beaten me. I'd told the hospital psychiatrist about sexual abuse, but no more. But I had never mentioned to a living soul that it was my father who'd been raping me. The memories of what he had done wouldn't stop haunting me.

I started to think that by telling someone, I might achieve release from the dark, haunting memories. The only person I could think of turning to was Felicity. She had become like a surrogate mother to me. I decided I would speak to her. One day after lessons I stayed behind with Felicity at college. I began to talk, and I told her some of what had happened, before I broke down in tears. I felt Felicity wrap her arms around me, warm and protective, as she hugged me and held me tight.

'Oh, Hannan, my poor dear. I love you. God loves you. You will get through all this, you will.'

I asked her not to tell anyone, but she told me that she didn't think she could keep it secret. She was my tutor and my guardian, and she felt that she had a responsibility to report what Dad had done. Knowing the depths of Dad's abusive ways, she was worried for my sisters' safety. I guessed she was right to be fearful. Sometimes I feared for their safety myself, especially now that I was gone.

'I'm afraid of going to the police,' I told her. 'I don't want to. I don't think I'm ready to tell them. I can't bear the idea of going into the detail they'll need. I just don't want to dig up all those horrible memories, especially with strangers.'

I knew what it would do to my family, and the community, if Dad was arrested for sexually assaulting his daughter. The shame of me running away from an arranged marriage would be nothing compared to that. An Imam being tried in a British court for raping his own child from the age of five to fifteen – it would tear the community apart.

What was more, I doubted whether the police would actually believe me. I was just a young girl and a college student. Dad was a pillar of the community. I remembered how Omer the social worker had immediately accepted Dad's word over mine. It seemed inconceivable to me that the police would hear me out, and believe me. It went against all that I had experienced and all that I knew. I explained all of this to Felicity.

'I understand your concerns,' she said. 'But how about if we talk to Barry? Maybe he'll know what to do. Would you be willing to do that?'

'Okay,' I said. 'I'll try.'

A day or so later I met up with Barry. He was such a kind, supportive presence that I was able to tell him some of what had gone on over the years. As he wasn't part of the child protection team, he had to refer me to them. A social worker from that team came to speak to me. Her name was Vicky, and she told me that I absolutely had to go to the police. I didn't see that I had much choice, so I agreed.

Vicky drove me to the police station. A woman officer took me into one of the interview rooms. We sat at a desk and she set a small tape-recorder running. She had a sheet of paper before her and a pen poised at the ready.

'Right, Hannan, tell me in your own words exactly what happened. Start with your name and where you used to live, and we'll go on from there.'

'My name is . . . My name is Hannan Shah. I . . . I . . . I . .'

I tried to get the words out, but I just seemed to freeze. My throat clammed up. I was unable to breathe almost. I started shaking, and I could feel tears welling up in my eyes. I was terrified about what might happen if I went ahead with this. I was terrified for myself. The physical act of forcing myself to talk made me panicky, especially with strangers. And I knew that if I went ahead with this statement it would launch a series of events that could never be stopped.

'I . . . I . . . I can't do this,' I managed to stammer. 'I just can't.'

The police lady seemed fine about it. 'If you're not ready, just come back when you are, okay? Don't worry. It's not a problem for us. We need you to be comfortable, and ready.'

I really needed that reassurance. It was crucial for me. I decided I would try to pluck up my courage for another day. Vicky, the child protection officer, said she would take me home. For a while we drove through the streets in silence. Then she gave me a sideways glance.

'Well, Hannan, you really messed up, didn't you? You were completely *useless* in there. You didn't tell them a thing. What a waste of everyone's time!'

I couldn't find the words to reply. I started crying and shaking again. All the way home she berated me for being so 'useless'. Once she'd dropped me off I called Barry. I told him what had happened, and what Vicky had said. Barry was enraged. He called up Vicky's supervisor and lodged a formal complaint. But the damage was done. I wouldn't be going to those child protection people again – at least, not for a very long time.

In due course the child protection team went to the primary

school to check on my little sister, Aliya. If there were any signs of abuse, or if the teachers had any concerns, they would put my sister on the 'at risk' register. Thankfully, there was nothing. I was so relieved. I didn't think that Dad would be doing the same to her as he had to me. To my knowledge, he had never beaten her. But I was still relieved.

And I was relieved not to have to take matters any further. In part, I was relieved for my own sake: I just didn't have the strength to go there. But it was also about protecting my family. Despite everything, I still cared about Mum, my sisters and my brothers. Reporting the abuse would be the beginning of the end for them all. It would hurl them into the abyss of torment, shame and dishonour.

As long as I thought my sisters were safe, the cost of going public about Dad was one that I really didn't know if I could inflict on my family. I didn't want them left without a husband and a father. However cruel and evil Dad was, trapped in our culture they would have been worse off without him.

A wife without a husband was nothing in our culture, and she would be prey to all kinds of prejudices and privations. Without their father, my sisters would have been equally vulnerable. I didn't want to see my family thrown to the wolves.

One day, Rachel and I went ten pin bowling with two guys from her youth group. It almost felt like a double date. One of the guys, Ian, was Felicity's nephew. He saw me again at my Bible study class on Sunday evening. After class, he came up to me.

'Hi, Hannan,' he said, nervously. 'Um . . . I really like you.'

I blushed. What on earth was he saying? I felt I was ugly and worthless. Everyone had always said so. What on earth could this tall, handsome, blue-eyed blond see in me?

'I'm going out with some of my mates on Tuesday,' he was saying. 'Would you come with me? Like on a date?'

'I'd like that,' I stuttered. I still couldn't believe what was happening.

He turned up that Tuesday evening and we walked to the

venue – bowling again. As we strolled along the street he reached out and held my hand. For an instant I almost drew it away. Being close to a man like this felt so odd to me, and would have been so frowned upon in my community. Doing such a thing on my street would have been an excuse for juicy gossip and scandal.

But I told myself to relax. I told myself to try to savour the moment. I knew it was innocent. There was nothing wrong in holding hands. In any case, as things turned out nothing more than holding hands would happen between Ian and me. We were hardly a match made in heaven. Ian was sweet, but he had a reputation for being a bit silly. He hadn't done well at school, and since leaving he'd had a string of part-time jobs. Now, he was drifting.

He did have one driving obsession, and that was football. It was to prove our undoing. Manchester United was his team, and I went with him to watch them play Southampton. During the match he started behaving oddly. Whenever his team scored a goal – and they scored four that day – Ian turned and hugged the girl on the other side of him. She was a white girl of about my own age, and she looked really shocked each time he did it.

I was confused myself. Had he forgotten which one of us he had come with? *Hang on*, I thought. *What are you up to? I'm right here!* I wasn't going to stand for this.

To get back at him I started shouting; 'Southampton! Come on, Southampton! *Southampton!*'

I hadn't quite realised that I was in the Manchester United stand, surrounded by their fans. But they soon realised what was happening. They found it hilarious whenever Ian hugged the wrong girl, and I cheered for the wrong team!

After the match Ian was really annoyed. As far as he was concerned cheering for the wrong side was the worst possible sin. But after his behaviour, what did he expect? I knew right then it wasn't going to work for me. I let the relationship die a natural death, and a while later I saw him holding hands with another girl.

I told Rachel and Zoë, and they looked a little guilty.

'Sorry,' said Rachel. 'I knew he was seeing someone, but I didn't want to say anything. I thought you might be upset.'

I laughed. 'Upset?' I exclaimed. 'Over Silly Ian? She can have him! I'm well out of that one.'

Shortly afterwards, Ian and his new girl got engaged. I wished them all the best, and I meant it, too.

I was studying and studying as hard as I could. When I finally sat my A-levels, I felt as if they had gone well. I decided that whatever my results, I would take a year off after college. I had been through an awful lot, and I felt I needed time to sort my life out before the challenges of university.

When the results came through, I had an A in Sociology, a B in Theology, and an E in English. I was ecstatic, and immensely proud. I knew I had done well enough to secure a place at university. In fact, I had exceeded the requirements set for me to take the Social Sciences degree at Lancaster University – the one to which I had applied. It was a dream come true.

That summer, the church youth group organised a trip to India. A group of us would visit a village in Tamil Nadu, a relatively poor state in the south of the country. It was a Hindu village, and we were going there to help build a well. It would mean four weeks abroad. I had only ever gone abroad once before, when I was three years old and my parents had taken me to Pakistan. It was an exciting challenge.

Our church had been allocated this village development project by a charity that worked all over India. Everyone who wanted to go had to raise enough money to cover travel and accommodation expenses, as well as their share of the costs of the well construction. We also wanted to buy textbooks for the village school. The target for each of us was to raise £1,500.

I did lots of different things to raise the cash – everything from washing cars at a church fete, to holding a talent show. At the church fete we had a stall where people could pay to 'gunge' someone – covering them in flour and eggs mixed with a blue dye, to make a big, slimy mess. Three people had 'volunteered' to be gunge candidates – myself, another member of the youth group, and pastor Bob. People paid money to vote for who they'd most like to see gunged out of the three of us.

There was no competition really. We three had to sit out front on plastic garden chairs while Felicity read out the votes. We all knew who was going to win – and sure enough it was poor pastor Bob! In no time he was covered in gunge, and everyone was cheering and laughing. It took him a very long time to get it all out of his hair.

It goes without saying, perhaps, that the very idea of my father – or any Imam for that matter – putting himself up to be 'gunged' was unthinkable. My father took himself and what he had to say far too seriously for that. It was a continuing revelation for me that religion could be *fun*. And I was so grateful that people from the church had clubbed together to help me raise the money to go to India.

Another thing I did to raise the cash was something I was uniquely qualified to do – I cooked a curry lunch! We planned to have the meal in the chapel, but just before it started something strange happened. Upstairs, there was an unstable wall that had been causing the churchwarden some concern. We had just come down from that room to have the curry when there was a huge crash upstairs.

Some of the adults ran back up to investigate. They came down a few minutes later covered in dust. The roof in the main chapel had fallen in, due to the unstable wall giving way. If we hadn't all just come downstairs for my curry lunch, the entire congregation would still have been up there. As it was, no one was hurt – so we decided we might as well carry on and tuck into the curry!

I had cooked chicken tikka masala, vegetable curry, rice and nan breads – going easy on the spices. The ingredients were donated by churchgoers, and others brought cakes and desserts. It was a real feast. There was a great atmosphere, and it was lovely for me to see people enjoying the food that I'd prepared.

Each person paid £5 for their curry lunch – so it was a bargain! Around 100 people turned up, so that event alone raised me £500.

By the time we were ready to go to India I'd raised £1,758 – more than enough to cover the trip. I had never been abroad on my own before, and I just knew the trip was going to be a real adventure. We arrived in the scorching heat of Tamil Nadu state, at the very southern tip of India. The villagers welcomed us with a Hindu ceremony, thanking the gods for the schoolbooks we had brought, and the well that we would build.

There was a small dam on a river that ran through the village, and on it they had placed a gold plate with candles and incense and jasmine flowers. There was a lot of singing and dancing. The sadhu – a holy man with wild, dishevelled hair, beads around his neck and a loincloth around his waist – chanted and led the Hindu prayers. And then the villagers asked us to reciprocate.

In spite of the poverty and deprivation that I saw, I loved my time in India. And I loved the fact I was doing something to help others, and disregarding my own situation. I loved learning about other people's lives, cultures and belief systems. Wherever I went, children would just run up to me and grab my hands and walk with me all through the village. I had never seen such free warmth and affection.

Each time I tried to pay the children back by teaching them an English rhyme.

> Round and round the garden,
> like a teddy bear,
> one step,
> two step,
> tickly under there!

On the last line I'd tickle their tummies. The kids loved it, especially the tickly bit!

Towards the end of the trip we took a few days off in the neighbouring state of Kerala. We spent a day on the beach, swimming and sunbathing. There was a bar-café run by a German man. As the day wore on he tried selling us some drugs, which turned out to be wraps of heroin. Then we spotted him giving some to the local children, which they had to sell to the tourists. You could tell that those children were drugged up: their pupils were dilated, and they acted strangely. It was horrible to see.

I felt so angry with the bar-owner. There was one little girl who looked to be round about six years old, but was probably older. She was so skinny and unwashed; it looked as if she had simply given up on life. Her lips were dry and cracked, and she wandered around vacantly. My heart went out to her. I went over and tried to give her a banana, but she just stared at me blankly. She wouldn't even take it. She was just empty, and there seemed to be no way that I could reach her.

I found that experience so disturbing. I wondered what had happened in her life, and where her family might be. I related to that girl and her life. I felt her trauma and her pain. I had spent my childhood alone and lost, giving up on life. No one was looking out for her – not even the other kids – just as no one had ever looked out for me.

I left India having seen so many people in need. The trip really served to put my own life into perspective. Yes, it had been tough. It had been hellish – a living hell at times. But there were even tougher places to be – like the place of that little, lost heroin-addicted girl on the beach. At least in England there were people who did come to my rescue – Mrs Zorba, Barry and Felicity. Who was going to help rescue *her*? Who was going to save *her* life and offer *her* sanctuary?

On a personal level, the trip gave me a lot of new confidence. The fact that I had done that journey on my own really built me up. When I got back home I gave a presentation for those who had helped me raise the money. I told them about where I had been and all that I had done. I even told them about the little girl on the beach. I would never have had the confidence to do that sort of thing before.

Bit by bit my life was getting better. While I was away, my friend Rachel had found me a lovely place to live. A family from the church had offered to rent me a room in their house. It was good to be back living with a family again, after my stint of going it alone. I'd had enough of that. I'd been hard on myself. Now I wanted a bit of company.

One day I went with Rachel to visit a church where she had some good friends. After the service I spotted an elderly white lady who looked somehow familiar. It suddenly came to me. It was Edith Smith, the woman who had come to our family home to teach Mum English all those years ago. I went up and introduced myself. Last time I had seen her I had been a six-year-old girl, but she did remember coming to our house.

She smiled at me. 'Yes, I do remember, you know. And your delightful mother, how is she?'

'Well, I don't have too much to do with her,' I explained. 'Mum's okay, I think. But I've become a Christian, so I have to keep a bit of distance.'

'How extraordinary! Well, you must come back to my house for tea. I'd love to hear all about it.'

With the sound of her voice, memories had come flooding back to me, by no means all of them pleasant ones. I remembered Mum and her in the lounge, laughing and joking about her pronunciation. But I also remembered Dad's savage beatings, and my intervention to try to save Mum, and the dark horrors that had followed.

'Mum isn't very well, unfortunately,' I explained. 'Her asthma is quite bad. I speak to my family on the phone quite a bit, but things are far from perfect, as you can imagine.'

I didn't say anything about the trouble and trauma her English lessons had led to in our household. I didn't mention Mum getting beaten up by Dad, or why Mum had stopped her from coming. I feared that it might upset her. And I certainly didn't want to say anything about how Dad had used her visits as an excuse to focus his violent and abusive ways on me.

In reality, Edith Smith wasn't responsible for what had

happened. The only person who was responsible for Dad's violence and sick behaviour was Dad.

Towards the end of my gap year I decided to get baptised. It was something I felt I had to do, to both celebrate and reaffirm my conversion. It was another step towards growing in my faith and celebrating my free choice as a free person in a free society.

I decided to invite my family to my baptism. I wanted them to see how important my newfound faith and identity were to me. I wanted them to recognise the freedoms that I was experiencing, having escaped from the ghetto of my street. At the service I planned to give testimony about how my life had changed. I wanted to talk about the joys of discovering who I was and what I could do with my life: speaking in public; raising money and going to India; studying hard and winning a place at university; and building real and meaningful friendships.

I hoped hearing all of that might open my family's eyes. What was more, I wanted to show them that, in spite of everything, I had forgiven them. I knew how important the concept of forgiveness was in my newfound faith, and it was something that I was determined to live by. I needed to explore forgiveness with my family. I wanted Mum to know that I forgave her. Inviting them to my baptism was a way of saying to them that they were forgiven. Well, apart from Dad. I didn't really know if I could ever forgive my father.

I knew that on one level I was being hopelessly naive in inviting my family. I knew that it might be foolhardy and even dangerous. At this stage, I had never heard of the word 'apostasy'. I didn't know that it says in the Hadiths (the collected traditions about what the prophet Mohammed said, did, permitted and prohibited) that anyone who converts out of Islam and refuses to return should be killed. I didn't know that converting out of Islam was considered one of the greatest sins of all. But even had I known this, I would probably still have invited my family. I wanted them to see where my life was going and where freedom's journey was taking me.

I rang up Billy. For a while we chatted about family and stuff, and then I decided to get on with it.

'Billy, you know I told you I'd become a Christian? Well, I'm going to get baptised. And I want you to come. It's something that's very special to me, Billy. I'd really like you to be there, and Mum and Raz and everybody.'

Billy just kind of snorted. Other than that, he didn't respond. Still, I went on to tell him the date and the place where I would be baptised. And then, after a second or so of silence, my nice brother Billy just put the phone down on me.

It was like a door had been slammed in my face. I was really, really upset, but I wasn't entirely surprised. *Well, there's my answer*, I thought to myself. *They're not coming.* Billy was the most liberal of the lot of them, so if that was his reaction I had no hope with the others. I took a deep breath, and decided to put it to the back of my mind. I'd tried. I'd done my best. There was nothing more I could do now.

A few days later I was alone in the house. It was mid-afternoon, and I was in my bedroom doing some studying. Suddenly I heard a wild commotion outside. I ran to the window. As I gazed down into the street I couldn't believe my eyes.

There before the house was a mob of around forty Pakistani men. They were armed with hammers, sticks and knives. Dad was at the front, his face a mask of hatred and fury. To my horror, even my 'liberal' Uncle Kramat was there, shouting and yelling wildly like the rest. I couldn't see any of my brothers, or any of the women from the street, but I didn't stay at the window to study the crowd in detail.

I rushed into the rear of the house to hide. I knew the front door was locked. But even so it was just a Yale lock, and with forty screaming men outside it could easily be smashed down. A few blows with their hammers and knives, and they would be in. I had a vision of the mob surging up the stairs, their weapons brandished before them, their eyes wild with hatred and blood lust. It was terrifying.

The uproar began.

'Filthy traitor!' Dad thundered. 'Traitor! Traitor! Traitor! You betrayer of your family! *Betrayer of your faith!* Cursed traitor! We're going to rip your throat out! We'll burn you alive!'

There was a pounding and a hammering on the door. I crawled further under the bed, shaking with fear, and I prayed to God to protect me.

I heard the letter box rattle, and suddenly Dad was screaming through it: 'Filthy, dirty traitor! TRAITOR! We're going to cut you up! Slice you! Burn you! Rip out your traitorous heart. Traitor – you'll rot in hell!'

I was utterly terrified. If Dad broke down the door and got his hands on me, I knew what was coming.

I would be beaten to death by the mob.

Chapter Twenty-two

The Mob

I was living in a white, working-class area, and I had no idea how my father had found me. But found me he had. For what seemed like an age the chilling, terrifying sound of hammers and sticks smashing on the door, plus the snarled curses and insults, and death threats, continued.

But all of a sudden it just went quiet. I lay there under the bed, barely daring to breathe. My heart pounded fearfully. What had happened? Had they gone? Were they inside the house, and sneaking up on me? Had they gone around the back to scale the garden fence? I just didn't know.

I finally plucked up courage to crawl out from under the bed. I crept forward to the front of the house. Still I could hear nothing. I reached for one of the net curtains, and jerked it back an inch or two. The entire street seemed deserted. Just as quickly as the crazed mob had come, they had disappeared.

I could only imagine that the locals must have come out onto the street. Maybe, for once in his life, Dad had realised that he wasn't going to have it all his own way. This was a tough, white working-class area. They wouldn't have taken kindly to their street being invaded by a screaming 'Paki' mob.

Or maybe my father had concluded that I wasn't in the house. All I had done was peep from an upstairs window. Most likely, I hadn't been spotted. Maybe he had been forced to conclude that he and his men were besieging an empty house. Maybe they had been forced to abandon the attack in frustration. But I also felt that my prayers had helped me. They had certainly given me strength.

Still, I was shaking uncontrollably. I knew I was lucky to be alive. I waited until I was certain the mob were gone. Then I dialled Rachel's number.

'Hello?'

'Rachel, it's Hannan,' I whispered, in a trembling voice.

'Hannan! What's wrong? Are you okay?'

'No. Yes. I mean – something terrible's happened. I'm really, really scared. I need your help, Rachel . . .'

'What?' I could hear the fear in her voice. 'What is it? What's happened? Tell me!'

I was worried that if I told her the threat that I faced from Dad and the mob, then Rachel wouldn't help me. I was worried that she would be too scared to come. In my panic, I told her the minimum I could to get her to come to my aid.

'Look, I can't talk over the phone. Can you come? I'm at the house. I need you, Rachel. I really do.'

'Of course. I'm on my way. Don't worry.'

I went and stuffed my few possessions into a bag. Five minutes later I heard a car pull up, and there was a knock at the door. I peeped outside. Relief flooded through me. It was Rachel's car. I ran out and dived inside.

We made straight for Rachel's house, and that's where I stayed that evening and for several days afterwards. I didn't tell Rachel and her family exactly what had happened. I just told them I had had a threat from my family, and I needed to get right away from the house.

I was shocked and very scared. I hadn't for one moment thought that Dad would react with such an extreme and public show of aggression and violence. Up to now the beatings and abuse had always been in secret. But suddenly, the violence was out in the open, and the community were right behind him.

All those faces of my family and relatives and the men from my street, twisted into masks of hatred. All of them threatening vengeance against me, and death. And all because I had dared to imagine that I was free to choose my own faith. They haunted my sleeping and my waking moments.

Still I went ahead with my baptism. Because my family knew which church I was planning to attend, I had to change the venue. Rachel pressed me to call the police and report Dad, but I resisted. The reasons were the same as before. I didn't want to be the focus of this battle. I just wanted to get on with my life, and to be left in peace. And I didn't want the implosion of my family on my conscience for the rest of my days.

Even so, my life had to change radically. I was in hiding now, and I would have to reconcile myself to having no more contact with my family.

A few weeks later I called Skip to ask her what was happening. Word had gone round about my father's rabble-rousing. Skip warned me that my family were looking for me, as was the entire street. I should be very, very careful. There was a dark anger simmering in the community over 'one of their own' leaving Islam. That's what had really got their blood up, especially with my father fanning the flames of their righteous rage. They knew that girls ran away. It happened. They knew young women fled from forced marriages. It happened. But leaving Islam – that was beyond the pale.

I was worried about Skip. My family knew she was my closest friend from the street, and they put her under a lot of pressure to tell them where I was. But rebel Skip wasn't about to tell them a thing. Quite the reverse, in fact. Whenever someone did find out where I was living, the buzz would go round the community. It was then that Skip would give me a warning call, and I'd pack my bag and go.

Luckily, I could always rely on my friends from the church to help me. I'd call them up and they'd come and fetch me, and take me somewhere where I could stay for a while. While they didn't understand exactly why it was so dangerous for me, they appreciated the urgency. They would drop everything and make sure I was relocated the very same day.

My family told Skip that I had to renounce my newfound faith. Otherwise they would not rest until they had hunted me down. I had to go back to them, and Islam, and marry the man they had chosen for me. It turned out that my suspicions had been correct. Mum's family had decided upon my birth that I would marry that distant cousin – the one whose photo I had been shown. If my father had succeeded in spiriting me onto that aeroplane, I would now be that man's wife. And most likely, I would be living in a remote Pakistani village surrounded – and imprisoned – by his relatives.

By now I had realised that for many Muslims apostasy was considered to be the greatest sin in Islam. I had woken up to the 'crime' that I had committed in the eyes of my community. I understood that was why my family were trying to hunt me down. I was shocked and deeply saddened by what had happened. I was also scared. But I didn't dwell on it.

I just wanted to put it all behind me, as I had done with everything else. It was too much to think about. It was emotional overload. All I wanted to do was stay hidden, and be free to get on with my life.

During the year after my father and the mob came to attack me, I was forced to move house every three months or so. I stayed with friends, families of friends, or in temporary rooms rented here and there. I was always ready to move at a moment's notice if I got warning that my family had tracked me down. I had one bag that I lived out of, and I could flee at any time.

I also anglicised my name from 'Hannan' to 'Hannah'. I didn't kid myself that that made it any harder to find me. I was living from day to day now, with no idea when I might have to move on. This hand-to-mouth existence made it all but impossible to plan things. I saw my dreams of going to university fading as the dangerous game of cat and mouse continued.

It was impossible to feel settled, or to put down any roots. It was impossible to study, or to hold down work for long. I felt as if I had physically escaped from my father, yet still he had found a way to keep my mind imprisoned in the nightmare.

I missed the chance to start studying for my degree that year. It wasn't until two years after the mob had come to attack me that I finally felt able to try again for university. During all of that time I had no contact with my family. But they were always there in my mind, like a dark shadow of blind prejudice and hatred hanging over me. I reapplied, this time to take Theology and Religious Studies, at Lancaster University.

I'd been advised that Lancaster University had a great Theology department, complete with top-class lecturers. I had always been fascinated by different belief systems, and I had loved the philosophy module in A-level Religious Studies. I had enjoyed the way it challenged my mind with free discussion and free thought. It was that which had first made me think that I'd like to explore further the world's major faith systems. Now, at Lancaster Uni I was going to get my chance.

My conversion to Christianity hadn't in any way diminished my fascination with other faiths and belief systems. I noticed that one of the options on the syllabus was 'Islamic Feminism'. Needless to say, I was fascinated by what that might be! And there were introductory courses to Judaism, Buddhism, and Hinduism, amongst other faiths. I wanted to study and to understand each of these more deeply.

I didn't really know what I wanted to do after university. I thought I might become a teacher, like Felicity, or a social worker, like Barry. These were the two people I most looked up to in my life. I knew I wanted to help young women who were trapped in a similar situation to the one that I had been in, and had yet to fully escape. I knew that the problems I had experienced were a growing issue. There were more and more stories appearing in the press about girls running away from arranged marriages, and about so-called 'honour killings'.

Skip would often call me with a report about another girl who had tried to escape her family's clutches. And then there were the young Muslim girls who would turn up at church, asking for help. On at least three occasions someone in our church found out about a girl facing a forced marriage. They came to me for advice, both on how to help, and how to make the family understand where the girl was coming from.

Some of the girls came from far more 'liberal' families than my own. On one occasion a young girl managed to talk to her folks and explain exactly how she felt. As a result, they cut a deal. The parents would allow her to go to university on the condition that they could revisit the issue of the arranged marriage once she had graduated. The girl seemed happy with that arrangement.

Sometimes, there was more openness in these families than at first seemed the case. All that was needed was dialogue and a little compromise on both sides. And that could stop it from ever reaching the stage where the immutables of 'honour' and 'shame' came into play. But they were the fortunate ones. And none of them was guilty of the ultimate sin – *apostasy*.

It was the Muslim network that was warning my family where I was living. Each Friday at the mosque my father would hand out a photocopied mug shot of me, with his phone number on the bottom of it. He asked people to ring him just as soon as they saw me. He may as well have been posting a wanted poster around my home town: 'WANTED: Hannan Shah. For the sin of APOSTASY'.

In that way my father created a network of spies to keep tabs on me. People would see me on the street, and that would pin me down to living in a specific area. With more sightings, he could narrow down exactly where my house might be.

I thought about moving away from the north of England altogether, to get away from my family and their spy network once and for all. But all of my friends were there. They were my new family, and I was loath to leave them. And it was at Lancaster that I had secured a place to study for my dream degree. Lancaster was a big, multi-ethnic city, I reasoned. I could sink into its vast urban anonymity, and forget all about my pursuers.

Surely to God I would be safe there.

Chapter Twenty-three

The Certainties of Ignorance

My first few days at university were ones of total freedom and release. I suddenly felt that it didn't matter what I wore, what I looked like, what colour my skin was, or what I believed. There were people there of every race, colour and creed imaginable. And there were people from every 'social tribe' ever invented – from Goths to Hippies to Sloanes and Rugger Buggers, and everything in between.

I made friends quickly. From the very start I hit it off with three girls from my course. They became my buddies, my gang, and we got a house to share in central Lancaster.

Anna was a white girl from Durham. She was short and a bit dumpy, with curly black hair. She had unrestrained, eclectic tastes, and was studying theology, philosophy and languages.

Tamsin was a white local girl. Tall, slim and exceptionally beautiful, she was the belle of the bunch. From day one she got chatted up the whole time. But the boys soon realised that she was a 'boring swot', and no party animal. In any case, Tamsin intended to marry her childhood sweetheart. She went for the more Biblical courses: the Old Testament, the New Testament, and Biblical Archaeology.

Then there was Jenny, another white girl, with light brown hair. Jenny came from Bury, and she wore flowing, flowery, hippie-ish clothes. She was the most creative of us all – a talented guitar player who loved writing and singing her own songs. Her interests lay chiefly in languages – Greek and Hebrew, plus an Urdu module that she and I both opted for.

And finally there was me. My hair was long and very curly, and at this point I'd put on quite a lot of weight. I didn't have the boys after me. I don't think I would have shown that much interest, anyway. On the rare occasion that someone did try to chat me up, they didn't get much of a response. I was too focussed on my studies, and hardly a very encouraging prospect!

Of an evening we four might go to the local pub, or to the Student Union bar. I'd realised by now that I really didn't like the taste of alcohol, so I was almost teetotal. The only alcoholic drink that I did like was Malibu and pineapple, but it was too expensive for me to buy it very often. A young man might just get a smile out of me if he offered to buy me a Malibu and pineapple though!

Our house was near Lancaster's famous curry quarter. Whenever it was a friend's birthday, we'd head to the curry quarter and try a different restaurant. But none of us were party animals exactly. All of us shared a desire to enjoy our studies and to do well. I guess we were all swots, really, and proud to be so!

I wasn't doing a course that required it, but one of the first things I decided to do at university was to read the Quran in English. After years of being told by holy men – like my father – what to believe, I just needed to see what it said for myself. As a child I had memorised many of the verses of the Quran in Arabic, yet without understanding more than a few words. Now I wanted to know the truth, and to understand.

I bought an English translation at WH Smith. I started reading it at home, in the evenings, after my lectures and homework were done. Sure enough, there *was* the wrath and anger that my father had vented on me at every turn. But there were also many more gentle, humane verses, including ones about giving money to the poor, and looking after widows and orphans. Why had my father never told me those? Not once did it say that alms should be extended only to fellow Muslims. The milk of human kindness was to be offered to whomever was in need, regardless of their race, colour or creed.

As I read the Quran for the first time and actually understood it, I began to realise that a lot of the things Dad had told me were in the Quran actually weren't there at all. Or at least I couldn't find them. And a lot of what was there had been twisted into a rigid creed of exclusion and control, seemingly at the whim of my father and his ilk.

This was the case even at the most basic of levels. For example, it doesn't say in the Quran how you should pray. There is no prescription as to the words or the actions required of a Muslim to pray. The ritual of standing, kneeling and bowing one's forehead on the ground facing towards Mecca doesn't appear anywhere in the Quran. The prayers are there as verses in the Quran, but nowhere does it say you have to pray using strictly those verses, five times a day, at specific times.

As far as my father was concerned, performing those five daily prayers was the very essence of Islam. Strict adherence to doing them was a Muslim's surest path to paradise. But where did it actually say that in the Quran? I couldn't find it anywhere, and in fact, these details are drawn from the Hadiths.

I read the Quran from cover to cover, and then I read it again. I was really angered when I discovered that there was nothing whatsoever in there about arranged marriages. Dad had told me repeatedly that the Quran said that every Muslim woman should have an arranged marriage, and that her parents should arrange it for her. In truth, there is not one single reference to this in the entire Quran. Indeed, the Quranic view of marriage involves a legal contract, with women having rights; she cannot be forced to marry against her will.

In fact, if you paid attention to the implicit lesson embodied in the life of the Prophet Mohammed, he married his first wife, Kadija, *for love*. She was a wealthy older woman who had been widowed. He was employed by her as a trader. In time *they fell in love*, and that was the reason they got married. Kadija wasn't related to Mohammed. In fact, they came from different tribes. So where on earth did the idea come from that young Muslim women should be forced to marry their cousins?

My father had insisted that was what it said in the Quran,

but it was a total lie. I could only imagine that it came from the indigenous traditions of my family's tribal area in Pakistan. There was not the slightest thing Islamic about it, or at least not as far as the Quran, the Muslim holy book, was concerned.

Other things amazed me. At its most basic, the Quran is Allah's word as revealed to his prophet, Mohammed. But it was not the story of Mohammed's life. It was a book of many stories: of Jesus' (Isa's) birth: of how the Angel Gabriel came to Mary (Maryam) and told her how Jesus was going to be born as a prophet sent by Allah. The story of Isaac and Ishmael, and the story of Abraham's (Ibrahim's) wife and her slave. The tales about Moses (Musa), Jacob (Yaqub), Joseph (Yusuf), and Job (Ayub).

There was a chapter entitled 'Women', about how Muslim women should be treated. It said that *both men and women* should dress 'modestly', and that women should be cherished and protected. It did say that husbands were allowed to 'beat' their wives for 'ill-conduct'. But there was nothing saying that women should be veiled from head to toe, and there wasn't one single mention of their hair and faces having to be covered. It just says that men and women should dress modestly.

So where on earth had all that come from? My father had insisted on all bodily flesh being covered at all times. We women always had to wear shalwar kamiz and a hijab. This was one of his most basic 'rules', and he enforced it because it was 'in the Quran'. Well, the truth was that it *wasn't* in the Quran. Not at all. There was absolutely nothing that said this at any stage in the holy book of Islam.

But some of the Surahs did surprise and disappoint me. Surah 2:223 said that a wife was 'tilth' for her husband: 'tilth' is ploughed land, ready for cultivation. The notes and commentary in the English version of the Quran that I was using interpreted this as meaning: 'You can have sexual relations with your wife in any manner, as long as it is in the vagina and not in the anus.' Other verses seemed to have other, equally misogynistic, bents to them.

On my second reading of the Quran I took to counting the number of mentions made of Jesus. There were actually ninety-five. By contrast, there were twenty-seven mentions made of Mohammed. So how on earth had my father been able to yell at me that I wasn't even allowed to 'mention' Jesus' name in our house? To me, this was nonsensical. The Quran spoke of Jesus being a healer, and it noted that he performed miracles. There was no mention of his supposedly pariah status, as decreed by my father.

I was drawn to one story in particular – that of Hagar and Ishmael. In the Old Testament it said that Abraham was asked to offer up his son, Isaac, for sacrifice. In the Quran, he is asked to offer up Ishmael. The Old Testament says that Isaac was the one chosen to carry on the line of Abraham – to create God's holy lineage. Isaac's descendants became the Jews. But the Quran maintains that Ishmael's line is the holy line, and that Mohammed is a descendant of Ishmael. It was Ishmael's descendants who founded the Muslim nation.

This story went to the heart of who was chosen by God to carry on the holy line – Isaac or Ishmael? The Jews or the Muslims? And that was a fine – some might argue *opaque* – dividing line. Many of the stories in each holy book had huge similarities between them: they shared characters, parables and messages.

The Quran was certainly *not* the Quran as taught me by my father. I spent hours and hours studying what it *was* about, and the Hadiths that accompany it. I payed particular attention to the issue of converting out of Islam – so-called apostasy. It did indeed say that a Muslim could kill a fellow Muslim if they turned away from Islam and refused to return (all be it after the due process of law was done).

But I didn't feel any more angry or scared than I had done before. I doubted whether my father actually knew any of this, bearing in mind some of his other glaring misapprehensions. The intention of the mob raised by my father had been crystal clear. I knew full well that this was what they were trying to do to me. I was certain that his desire to kill me – and the blood lust that he had whipped up within the community – was more about the community's traditions of honour and shame.

Prior to reading the Quran, I had never really questioned whether my father knew his holy scriptures. If he didn't, how could he be a religious leader – an Imam – I had reasoned. I had presumed that what he had taught me was Islam. Now I knew the truth. Very little of his most dogmatic beliefs and blind prejudices were actually in the holy book of Islam. For him to say these things, and to claim they were in the Quran, constituted a level of ignorance, arrogance and hypocrisy that was breathtaking. It was also sacrilege.

Of course, other Imams in the sort of community that I came from would reinforce what he believed to be true. Many were saying the same kind of things. You'd have to have real courage and guts to examine it for yourself, and to stand up for truth and for your own religion. In any case, in the culture of my father's generation you never questioned your elders or teachers. Religious learning was based around an oral tradition, where things were passed down and learnt by rote.

The potential for a 'Chinese whispers' effect, where misrepresentations got magnified time and time again, was immense. At first the truth would be denied. Over time, the truth would be forgotten. Finally, the misrepresentation would become the accepted version of the truth.

But none of this was an excuse, of course. I was angry at my father, and I was angry at those like him. What on earth were some young Muslims in Britain – and elsewhere – being taught? No doubt much the same as I had been – my father's brand of Islam. So much of that was opinionated, prejudiced rubbish, very little of which was in the Quran.

For the first time in my life I had a much clearer view of Islam, and I didn't believe my father's version any more.

I started having discussions with Muslim students on my course about what I'd read. I asked them what they thought about the ninety-five mentions of Jesus, or the whole chapter on Mary, his mother. More often than not they seemed not to know of such things. So, I'd quote them chapter and verse, and they'd promise to go away and look it up. It turned out that most of them had never read the Quran, except in Arabic. Like everyone else from my street, they didn't know what it actually said. It was mind-boggling.

They came from the same generation and type of background as me, so I was half expecting this to be the case. That's why I was probing and asking such questions. Here were young, educated Muslim men and women in their twenties, studying theology at one of the UK's best universities for that subject. If even they were ignorant of what the Quran actually says, I could only imagine what the rest of the Muslim population might be like.

But what truly amazed me was that they hadn't come here to study or learn about their own religion, Islam, via a fuller understanding of the Quran. They seemed content to believe what they had been told – that it was somehow wrong to read it in anything other than the original, incomprehensible Arabic.

As for the lecturers, they appeared to be scared of making any critical appraisal of the Quran, or of Islam in general. Whenever I provoked discussion, a number of the Muslim students would get very upset and annoyed. They seemed unable to accept anyone questioning the meaning or interpretation of their holy book. And the lecturers seemed more inclined to defend this viewpoint than challenge it.

In the Islamic Feminism course I pointed out that the Quran says nothing about women needing to be veiled.

'Yes, it does!' one of the Muslim students retorted. She herself was wearing a hijab. 'Anyway, how would you know? You're not a *Muslim*. You're a *Christian*. How can you presume to interpret *our* holy book?'

'Have you ever read your holy book in a language that you understand?' I asked her.

'Well . . . No. But I'm not supposed to . . . It's only meant to be read in classical Arabic. It's not like the Bible, is it?'

'Well, I have read it – in English,' I continued, 'my native language. So, I do know what it says. Look up Surah 24:31. There it says that women should draw their veils over their bosoms, but it doesn't say anything about covering the hair or the face. And men are cautioned to "dress modestly", just as much as women are. So if a woman has to wear a veil, so should a man.'

The angry young woman flushed red with embarrassment. What could she say? She didn't actually know what was said in the Quran, so how could she even discuss it with me?

In arguments like this the Muslim students seemed ashamed when confronted by their ignorance of their own holy scriptures. As for the lecturers, they appeared uncomfortable when these topics were raised. They were teaching us about the writings of feminist Muslim writers, yet they didn't want to get involved in studying the Quran itself. It was almost as if the Quran alone amongst holy scriptures was beyond scrutiny or reproach.

I started talking privately with some of the more curious of the Muslim men and women on my course. We discussed what it said in the Quran, and I would point them to specific verses. Some of them went away and read them, and then we would continue our discussions. A number came back to me and admitted that, to their surprise, the Quran actually didn't say what they had been led to believe it did.

'You're right,' one young Muslim girl confided in me. 'There is no admonition to keep our faces covered. But it does say to dress modestly. Look at Surah 24:31.'

'That's true, but look at this Surah.' I had my English Quran with me, and pointed out the verse. 'Look – it clearly says that men *and* women should dress modestly. So surely if women veil, men should too, shouldn't they?'

One man did try to argue that for a woman, beauty is vested in her hair and chest, and a man didn't have the same attractions that needed to be covered. And the face, I asked him? How about that? He couldn't answer me.

I could see the confusion among the young Muslims who actually went away and read the Quran in English. It shook their certainties. But most refused to engage with me in any way at all. They persisted in reading the Quran in Arabic only. They chose to keep their minds closed. They seemed more comfortable with the certainties of ignorance, and I suppose it was their right to remain ignorant if they so chose.

None of them ever admitted to me that it was my reading the Quran in English – an activity that they had previously considered as spiritually derelict – which had given them the strength to do so. None of them said that my reading of it in English had implanted the idea in their minds. Yet I know that this was the case. Once again, my rebel spirit had proven that it would not be constrained.

The very word Islam means 'submission'. To many the very substance of what the faith has become is submission to the word of Allah, read in a language very few of the believers understand. The very idea of questioning anything within their received version of Islam was deeply shocking to these students. That was clear to me now. The Quran does speak of being a 'slave of Allah'. And perhaps slaves are not supposed to question, or even at times understand, their masters.

I had a tense relationship with the Muslim students, one that was largely about debate. Their attitude was a mixture of respect, because I could quote chapter and verse from the Quran, tinged with suspicion. Why was I asking these questions of their faith? Who was I to question what the Imams taught as truth and what they believed? A number of the male students were angry with me, and did little to hide that anger. They just told me that the Quran was the holy word of God, and as such should never be questioned.

'I'm not saying you should question the holy word of God,' I'd counter. 'I'm just saying you should read it in a language you understand. Surely it is better to believe from a position of knowledge, rather than one of ignorance? It has to be better to believe because you have read your holy scripture and understood it, rather than just listening to what other people tell you to believe?'

That didn't always go down so well. In their eyes, it was dangerous heresy.

Chapter Twenty-four

Hunted

At university I had hoped that the game of cat and mouse with my family had finally come to an end. But sadly, as I approached my final year I got another warning from Skip. Not for one moment had my family stopped looking for me, and somehow, Dad had found out where I was studying. I resolved to be more vigilant, and I hoped that my father's reach didn't extend into Lancaster's heart of academia.

One morning shortly after Skip's call I arrived at college on the bus. As I went to get off, I saw a familiar figure standing by the university gates. It was my brother Raz. I knew he had to be waiting for me. This confirmed Skip's warning. My family had indeed found me.

The shock of seeing Raz there really hit me hard. I had seen Lancaster University, and academia as a whole, as my inviolable sanctuary. It had been my place of freedom from my family and my dark past. Now that illusion had been shattered. After two years of living a relatively normal life, I knew that I would have to move house right away. Who could tell how much my family knew about me already? I would have to recommence my restless, nomadic existence.

I pushed back past the other passengers and stayed on the bus. I glanced out of the window to see if Raz had spotted me. He gave no sign that he had. He was still casting his eyes around, searching for a familiar figure amongst the throngs of students streaming into campus. I kept my head down as the bus pulled away. My heart was beating fast, and fear was once again coursing through my veins.

I got off at the next stop and phoned a close friend. Would it be possible to stay with her for a few days? I had to finish my degree, and I wasn't prepared to let my family ruin all that. I could go back to my nomadic lifestyle if I really had to. Above all else, I couldn't let them win.

Later, I sneaked back into college using a rear entrance. I went directly to speak to my lecturer in philosophy, Dr Law. He was in his early forties, and I liked and trusted him. Over the years we had had many interesting discussions about faith, tribe and identity. He knew that I'd converted out of Islam and that I had no contact with my family. I told him what had happened. Dr Law notified the administration department not to give out any of my details to anyone. Security were told to be extra vigilant.

The next day I discovered a note in my pigeonhole. It was from Raz. That really brought the threat home to me. This was how close they had got to me.

This is a note from your brother, Raz. You must get in touch.
We really need to speak to you. This is my number.

How had they tracked me down? I called Skip, and everything became suddenly very clear. Jamila, one of the Muslim women on my course, had become a friend of sorts. She was one of the people that I had engaged in conversation – or tried to – about the Quran. In fact, Jamila had been very closed to all of that. She had never gone away to read the Quran in English. Instead, we had found some common ground talking about Bollywood movies, the charts, and whatever was on TV.

What I had failed to realise – and what Jamila had never told me – was that she lived on the same street where Raz now ran a shop. Through Raz, Jamila had met my family. It was she who had told them that I was on the same course as her at Lancaster University. Just as soon as Skip had put me in the picture I confronted Jamila on the campus.

'I hear you told my family where I'm living. Why did you do that?'

Jamila looked worried. She tried to avoid any eye contact. 'Look, I just ran into your brother at his shop, that's all. He knows my uncle, and I knew they were looking for you, so I just thought I should tell them. What's so wrong . . . ?'

'Do you have any idea what you've done?' I cut in. 'Have you any idea how dangerous this is for me?'

'What do you mean? It's got nothing to do with me.'

'Nothing to do with you! Let me tell you – it is now! You've got yourself involved by telling them where I live.'

I turned my back on her and stalked off. After that, we never once spoke again, not even to pass the time of day. Her behaviour was selfish and unforgivable. I was furious. She had betrayed me. She had acted as if she was my friend, and then reported me to my family. Maybe she didn't know how dangerous it was for me. But she could have spoken to me first, and then I would have told her.

I didn't make contact with Raz. I was too scared to do so. I didn't know why he had come, but my last contact with my family had been watching a lynch mob, led by my father, coming to kill me because I was a 'traitor' to Islam. I had no desire for a repeat performance.

Raz was seen on the campus quite a few times, but no one could do much about it. It was a public space and unless some-one was in breach of the peace, he or she had a right to walk around more or less wherever they chose to. I didn't think Raz's intentions were necessarily bad or dangerous. By and large he was a gentle soul. But he was an instrument of my father, and him I truly feared.

The naïve hopes about a family reunion that I had nurtured at the time of my baptism had long since faded. But I did regularly pray for my family, and I hoped that in time they would come to an understanding of why I had chosen the path that I had. I prayed for Mum, that she would be well, and that my sisters would be happy. I prayed for reconciliation with my brothers. And from time to time I even prayed for deliverance for my father.

*

I used the end-of-term vacation to go to work for a Christian charity, in Greece. Each year, they hired a resort for a season, running holidays for Christian families. I was taken on as a youth worker. At least my family wouldn't be tracking me down there any time soon. I loved every minute of it, and I really hit it off with one particular family. They hailed from the upmarket southern English town of Farnham.

Talking to them made me think about escaping properly. They rarely got the chance to meet someone from my background, because there were so few Asians in Farnham. I felt as if my family were only ever one step away. The only way to truly break free had to be to get out of the north of England completely. I had to move somewhere where I wouldn't always be stumbling into people with links to my community and my past.

It was a hard thing to contemplate, for it would mean breaking so many ties to friends and community, but it was a move that I forced myself to think about seriously. Once I had graduated, perhaps I could head to Farnham, and really get away. With my brother stalking the college grounds, it was time to make a move. I decided that just as soon as I had graduated I would do so.

I finally graduated with a 2:1. I was immensely proud of what I had achieved. I had studied so hard and felt I really deserved my degree mark. It was sad that I couldn't share my success and happiness with my family, but there it was. Felicity was ecstatic. She, Zoë, Rachel and I went out to celebrate, having a slap-up meal at an Italian restaurant. Felicity told me she was so proud of me. It had been one hell of a journey from the day that I had run away from home, to here.

During my final term I had applied for several jobs in Farnham. The YMCA came through with an offer of accommodation and a living wage, if I would come and work for them. I jumped at the chance, and headed for the sunny south of England.

Farnham was the first place I had lived where there were few or no Pakistani Muslims. At first it was really weird. I walked down the high street and didn't see one Asian face. Nearly everyone was white. It was hugely noticeable to me, but no one seemed to pay me much attention. For the first time in my life I felt like I could disappear among the crowd.

The anonymity of being in a big southern English town made me feel safe. I didn't need to keep looking over my shoulder wondering if my family were following me, and about to get me. I'd lived with that feeling of being hunted for six years or more. Suddenly, the fear and the uncertainty were no longer there.

Of course, I was still suspicious of people. When I first met someone new in Farnham, I wouldn't tell them where I lived. It took me months to learn to trust people, and to relax my vigilance.

My work with the YMCA was chiefly in schools, helping with Religious Studies lessons. But I also had to help any homeless people who came into the hostel. I had to teach them a little independence, so they could move on with their lives. I found I could really relate to those who came in off the streets. Most, if not all of them, were running from something or other. And I felt that their situation was not so different from how I had spent my last few years.

Now I was living in Farnham I finally felt as if the running was over. There was no one from my street, or my community, to keep an eye out for me. At times I'd find myself panicking: *I've been here too long! I have to get on a train and move on, or else they'll find me!* But then I would take a deep breath, and tell myself that here I was safe. I didn't have to keep phoning Skip to find how close they had got to me, and planning my next move.

I knew that here I should be able to put down some roots at last. I enrolled on a PGCE course to train as a teacher. I moved into a house with some friends from my new church. But as my fear of my family finding me gradually subsided, the loss of them started to hit me hard. I missed my little sister, my brother Billy, and my mum. I wondered what they were doing now. The fear of being hunted had been replaced by a deep and residing sense of loss.

And when I stopped running physically, I realised that I had to stop running psychologically too. I could no longer hide from the sexual abuse that I had suffered. I knew that the time had come to face up to it.

It was time to walk into the darkness and banish it once and for all.

Chapter Twenty-five

Finding Me

Coming to terms with the sexual abuse that had poisoned the first sixteen years of my life was a daunting prospect. I still felt at this stage that it was partly my fault. What had I ever done to stop my father? I hadn't run. I hadn't told anyone. I still carried the shame. I felt as if every other relationship in my life was based upon a lie. When my friends told me that they loved me, I couldn't stop myself from thinking: *but would you really say you loved me if you knew it all?*

For years after it ended the abuse had made me feel disgusting, worthless and guilty. That damage didn't simply go away. The fact that I had hidden it for so long made me feel shame and guilt for having done so. It was my dirty little secret. I had told the whole truth only to God. Him I had been honest with, and thank God he hadn't rejected me.

In Farnham I met a girl called Samantha, and we soon became best of friends. Samantha was very much a cool extrovert. She was laid-back and bursting with energy at the same time. She was petite, with dark hair and dark, smoky eyes. She was great fun to be with. What was more, she had a huge heart. There seemed to be no limit to her ability to give.

We met at church, and in no time Samantha had enveloped me with her love. She invited me home to meet her family. Over time, they seemed almost to 'adopt' me as one of their own, rather as Felicity had done. I moved into a rented house with Samantha, and her brother, Chris. For the foreseeable future this was my permanent, safe home.

Samantha was arty and creative. There was a wooden shed in

the back garden. She decided that she wanted it as her bedroom. She liked the bohemian ambiance of the shed. It had electricity, so she had light and a heater. She could use it as her artist's studio, without ponging out the house with smelly paints. So Samantha's bedroom became the wooden shed in the garden.

Samantha, Chris and I lived together like a little family. We didn't have a cupboard each for food, as my university friends and I had done, and we cooked for each other. I was forever making spicy curries, which Samantha and Chris devoured. Samantha loved cooking chorizo and rich, Spanish dishes. And Chris did a passable pasta.

In the garden there was an orchard. Samantha decided she wanted to collect the apples to make apple crumble. She was so enthusiastic picking all the apples that no one had any energy left afterwards to cook. In the end, we went around the street giving the apples away. The next apple season we picked them all to make cider, and the same thing happened again. It was a second autumn that the people on our street really got to enjoy our apples.

Samantha was a dreamer, but in the nicest possible way. If she met a homeless person on the street, she would bring them home, cook a meal for them, and give them somewhere to sleep. She knew it wasn't fair billeting complete strangers in the house, so they'd usually end up in the garage. She even got into trouble with the church, because she let a homeless person sleep there one night. They had been holding a sleepover for kids when this homeless person had wandered in.

'Well, now you're here you may as well stay!' Samantha had told him, cheerfully.

So the homeless stranger slept the night in the church with the kids. No one seemed to appreciate it very much, and the church-warden was furious. But I loved her sense of spontaneity and generosity, and I respected her for how much she cared. Yet there was also a part of me that worried for her safety. In the middle of the night if she saw someone covered in blood after a fight, she would go to them and try to help. She was absolutely fearless, but she was tiny, and she would often be on her own.

I'd never met anyone like Samantha before, or even imagined that someone like her could exist on this earth. She acted as though she could never be hurt, as if no one would ever try to hurt her. But I feared that one day someone would turn on her, and that would change her attitude for ever. I worried about her ability to protect herself, and her wonderful, magical innocence.

I never wanted anyone to steal Samantha's innocence, as mine had been stolen as a child. But I guess Samantha had an angel looking over her shoulder, for she was never hurt for all her acts of heartfelt kindness. And Samantha was truly an angel towards me.

With the feeling of security that came with my new life, I guess I let my defences down. I started having nightmares and flashbacks to the darkest hours of the abuse – things that I had kept long buried. At times, Samantha sat up with me all night long. I was too scared to fall asleep again, in case I was dragged back into the darkness of the nightmare. Samantha was my rock at this time. It was a lot to ask of someone, to stand by me. Often, I used to wonder what she got from our friendship.

Samantha came from a very conventional, conservative English family, though she herself was thoroughly unconventional. Perhaps in me she had found someone with whom she could air her most unconventional ideas. She knew I would never judge her. I came from such a different background to the middle-class white friends she was used to. I carried none of their baggage into our friendship. And I always offered her an honest answer.

These days I didn't pull my punches, not with anyone. For so long I had lived in a community ruled by half-truths, opaque traditions and the strictures of 'honour' and 'shame'. My community had nurtured and maintained those 'rules' – reinforcing them, policing them, and feeding them on to others. I couldn't bear for my own life to be like that. I had to draw a line in the sand. I had to tell the truth, and hope that people would take me as I was.

I even found the little lies of southern English 'politeness' difficult. In Farnham, people were so polite they wouldn't ever tell you what they really thought. The only way I could deal with this was total honesty. If someone asked me what I thought of what they were wearing, I'd tell them – even if I thought it looked atrocious. It didn't always seem to go down so well.

But Samantha liked my honesty. She seemed to value getting a genuine answer, as opposed to the polite one. In this way, Samantha got something back from me, something she needed. But it was nowhere near what she offered me in our friendship, and what I was glad to accept from her.

I was plagued by those recurring nightmares, and when Samantha had sat up with me half the night I felt the least she deserved was my honesty. And so I revealed to her the full horror and the darkness that they contained. Samantha would react by holding me tight to her for hours on end, as if that might take away the pain and hurt. Sometimes she would cry with me, but most of the time she was strong.

I told Samantha more than I had ever told anyone. I trusted her with everything. I knew that I could trust her with my life. Samantha heard it all.

One day I went into Farnham town centre to do some shopping. All of a sudden I found myself in an area that I'd never seen before, wandering around lost and confused. In fact, hours had gone by without me realising. I was in a complete daze. I had my mobile phone with me, and I used it to call Samantha. She could tell that I was disorientated and scared. She asked me to describe the buildings I could see. Finally she worked out where I was.

'Sit tight!' she said. 'I'm coming to get you!'

She soon turned up and took me home. I had absolutely no idea what had happened. I had lost three hours or more. They were a total blank. I had no memory whatsoever of where I had been or what I had done. It was terrifying. I put it down to exhaustion and just having a 'funny turn'. But over time it started happening to me more and more often, and always, Samantha was there for me.

Samantha and I started to worry that there was something

going on medically, or psychologically – something that we didn't understand and couldn't deal with alone. Perhaps I needed professional help, Samantha suggested. Was the dark depression that had taken me into the psychiatric hospital coming back to haunt me again, but manifesting itself in a new and frightening way? I just didn't know for sure.

I went to see my GP and told him what had happened. He diagnosed depression, and prescribed me medication. But I was very reluctant to take the pills. To my mind, if I was depressed then there had to be a reason for me being so. Taking pills might treat the symptoms, but not the cause.

In our part of Farnham there weren't enough therapists to provide support to everyone who needed it, my GP explained. In fact there was a two-year waiting list to see one. In the meantime, the only option he could offer me was the drugs.

I decided that was something I didn't want. I opted instead to try a private, faith-oriented counselling service. The counsellors talked to me about my past; about the nightmares and the insomnia; and about the blackouts wherein I was losing myself for hours on end. Slowly, I began to open up about the worst aspects of the abuse. Finally, I even went into what happened to me in the cellar.

'Hannah, I'm starting to think you may be suffering from PTSD,' remarked my counsellor.

We'd been talking for several months now and I had really grown to trust her.

'What's PTSD?' I asked.

She explained that PTSD stands for 'post-traumatic stress disorder'. Soldiers who have seen awful things often find themselves suffering from PTSD. In fact, anyone exposed to extreme trauma can suffer from it – policemen, firemen, and even the victims of violent crime.

On the one hand it sounded so serious. *PTSD*. It was a label. Did it mean that I was really ill? But over time I found it useful to be able to define what was happening to me. Luckily, the vicar of my church had prior experience with PTSD sufferers – most of whom were British soldiers. He was a great support to me. In my case, the abuse had gone on for so long and was so deeply buried that there were other complications as well. But the immediate issue was the PTSD.

I took my 'diagnosis' back to my GP. He agreed that I might indeed have PTSD. All my symptoms fitted the diagnosis. At this point, he stopped trying to push pills on me. Only by talking and dealing with the trauma can a PTSD sufferer be cured. Eventually, I decided I wanted to cure myself by understanding what I had been through, and dealing with it accordingly. I put together my own treatment regime.

I found out about a retreat in the Cotswolds, called Harn Hill. It is a place of total peace, set among green hills, with sheep and cows grazing in the fields. It is a faith-based healing centre, where people sit together and talk through the trauma they have suffered. They would pray together, and meditate upon it. It was a place where one could do so in total peace and serenity, far removed from everyday life.

My first week at Harn Hill was a magical experience. I started to spend time there whenever I could, seeking the peace and the space to deal with my past. By talking about what had happened and putting it out in the open, I found I could slowly release the hurt and the pain. That, and the counselling, helped enormously. I felt myself becoming well again, to the point where I felt I was ready to forgive the guilty party – my father.

I didn't want to spend the rest of my life feeling like a victim, and being defined by the harm that he had done to me. I wanted to move on to a place where I could speak out about what had happened to me. I wanted to let go of the hurt and the hatred and resentment, for if I didn't it would only consume me.

And I also wanted to get over my distrust of men. Only then might I stand a chance of finding a man that I could love, and who could love me back in turn. As I felt myself becoming whole again, there was just one part of me that still felt empty.

That was the part of me that wanted to find love.

Chapter Twenty-six

Finding Love

On Christmas Eve 2006, I was at St Bride's Church, in Farnham. It was midnight mass, and I was one of those chosen to give a reading. The service was almost over when a young man turned around and started staring at me. For a moment I caught his eye, but then I looked away again just as quickly. What was he starring at, I wondered.

He didn't seem able to stop staring. It was unnerving, and rude, I thought. When the service finished, he hurried off to speak to a mutual friend of ours, called Jenny. I was glad that was over with. But unbeknown to me he was making further enquiries!

'*Who* is that beautiful girl?' he demanded of Jenny.

'Which beautiful girl?' Jenny countered. 'There's quite a few here tonight, or hadn't you noticed?'

'That one,' he replied, Jenny's teasing going completely over his head. 'The one who gave the reading. The one with the big brown eyes and gorgeous hair and . . .'

'All right, all right,' Jenny stopped him. 'I know who you mean. It's Hannah. Come on, I'll introduce you.'

Jenny and this strange man made their way over to me. She introduced him: his name was Tom. Jenny explained that she thought Tom and I should meet because I was a convert from Islam, and Tom was fascinated by Islam. But of course, it wasn't that at all. She was just trying to match-make. Almost immediately Tom started gabbling on about this and that, and an instant later he was asking for my phone number. I'd rarely seen such desperation in a man!

244

I told Tom I wasn't going to give him my number. I thought he was a bit forward just demanding to have it, and so quickly. Apparently, when he had seen me giving the reading, Tom was mesmerised. He decided there and then that he just had to get to know me better, whatever the cost. Little did he know what a tough nut I would be to crack.

I have to admit I was struck by what gorgeous blue eyes he had. He was 'arty'-looking, with a floral shirt and a goatee beard. He wasn't the sort of guy I would normally go for, but he was miles better-looking than Ian – my date from all those years ago who was obsessed with Manchester United. Still, I didn't believe that Tom had *romantic* interests. And even if he did, he didn't half seem weird. Why did I always seem to attract the oddballs, I wondered.

Tom wasn't put off by the lukewarm reception. Instead, he just talked Jenny into handing over my number. The next day he called me up out of the blue. He had tried to get to Jenny's house for Boxing Day, for he knew that I was going to be there with Samantha and some other friends, but he hadn't made it. So he called instead.

'Hi, it's Tom. Remember me? From the church . . .'

'Yes . . . Kind of,' I replied, cautiously. 'How on earth did you get this number? I seem to remember refusing to give it to you.'

'I'll tell you how I got your number if you let me come round to visit you later today, okay? Deal?'

I had to give him ten out of ten for perseverance. Samantha and Chris would be in the house, so I didn't see it could do any harm. And anyway, a small part of me was intrigued. Just who was this Tom guy? And what harm could it do to let him visit? At least I'd find out which of my friends had given out my number. I was certain it had to be Jenny. There was a real mischievous streak in her, which I adored.

'Can I come round to see you?' Tom prompted.

'Fine. Okay. Come round for tea or something . . .'

A few hours later Tom turned up at our house. He spent an hour sitting on our couch, babbling on about Lord only knew what. He was a whirlwind of words and nervous energy. He kept asking me question after question, without giving me any time to answer. He hardly seemed to register that Samantha and Chris were there.

By the time he left I was none the wiser about what he'd been going on about. It had all been so jumbled. I thought to myself: *What an oddball! I'll just have to hope he keeps out of my way.*

Jenny called later. 'So? *So?* What d'you think of Tom then?'

'Tom? *Tom.* I think he's a bit of a babbling idiot, to tell you the truth. Thanks, Jen, but from now on try to keep him away from me, will you?'

Jenny cracked up laughing. 'Come on, don't be too harsh. Poor Tom. He's not that bad. He's got gorgeous eyes . . .'

Still Tom didn't give up. His next approach was via text messaging:

Please come and see me in Southampton.

The community. We need it.

There's lots of Muslims here. Tom.

Sorry? What? What on earth was that all about? It left me absolutely none the wiser. I just texted back, saying:

OK. I'll come when I find the time.

I was actually very busy with work, and it was hard to find time out for anything, let alone oddball Tom. I had started running a series of workshops about Islam and cross-cultural issues. It was part of my work with a tiny charity called Crossways. Crossways helps people from different backgrounds to better understand Islam – both the belief system and the culture that so often goes with it.

I ran the workshops for Muslim girls focussing on how to communicate with their parents on issues like arranged marriages, and other problems they might face. The aim was to get dialogue going, before 'shame and honour' came into the equation.

At one of those workshops who should turn up but Tom. He wandered in and told me right away how fascinated he was by the issues I was raising. He had come to listen and to learn. He was almost an hour early and he tried to help me set up. But he was all fingers and thumbs, and he just got in the way. He hung around right to the end, whereupon he didn't seem to want to leave.

'Tom, you really do have to go,' I told him, eventually. 'I have to pay for this hall by the hour. You've got a minute to make yourself scarce, *or you're paying!*'

I offered him a lift to the train station, just to get him out of the way. My boss at Crossways thought he knew exactly what was going on. He kept telling me that Tom fancied me.

'That's impossible,' I'd say. 'He's just fascinated by Islam and stuff. Anyway, I hope not. I always end up with the odd ones . . .'

At the next workshop Tom was there again. I was giving a talk on clothing, and I had turned up wearing shalwar kamiz.

Tom gazed at me and smiled shyly. 'You look . . . serene,' he remarked, dreamily. 'Just so serene.'

I wasn't quite sure what he meant by that, but I smiled politely. At least the shalwar kamiz wasn't canary yellow!

There was a piano at the back of the hall, and rather than getting in the way of me Tom sat down at it. He opened the keys, and suddenly he just started to play. He chose a song by Jamiroquai, and he played it entirely from memory. As his hands flashed over the keys I stared at the back of his blond head, the music flowing from him like magic. Tom played beautifully, like a wild and blazing angel. I was captivated.

As soon as he stopped playing the spell was broken, but for a moment there I had seen another side of Tom, and it was a side that I could maybe . . . like. I turned away, and a thought came unbidden into my mind: *okay, maybe I need to give this guy a chance.* As Tom had worked his magic over the piano's keys, I had been able to study him a little more closely without being babbled at. He was actually a fine-looking young man.

Perhaps sensing the change in me that his piano playing had wrought, Tom invited me to have a day out with him in Southampton, where he lived. This time, I accepted, and we had a wonderful time together. Once Tom had relaxed a little and got over being tongue-tied, he was great company.

'Why not come and visit my church?' Tom asked me, shyly. 'Come and meet my friends. I'm sure they'd love to hear all about your life.'

'Okay,' I replied, with a smile. 'Why not?'

But I had only agreed because I wanted to see Tom again.

'And, erm, would you like to have dinner tonight?' Tom added.

'Sure! Sounds great. I'd love to.'

Unfortunately, on the way to the restaurant Tom seemed back to his babbling self. I wondered why? When we sat down to eat, I found out. He had been trying to pluck up courage to tell me how he felt about me.

'Hannah, I think you're hot,' he blurted out. 'You're a real babe! I really want to go out with you.'

I smiled. 'All right . . . Well, let's take it slowly and give it a try.'

That was in May. By that summer Tom and I were inseparable.

I was forever asking Tom about life, belief, and how he dealt with pain, and painful situations. There was a struggle within me, as I suspect there is in every one of us, over how to deal with pain and hurt. On the one hand, you could shrivel into bitterness and recrimination. On the other you could rise above all that, and take the risk once more to engage with the beauty and unpredictable, intoxicating riot of life.

You could choose to risk life throwing whatever it might at you, and acknowledge that pain and hurt are possible, but knowing that with these come love and the joy and the richness of human experience. I was determined to do the latter, and especially so in my relationship with Tom.

I had 'The Invitation' by Oriah Mountain Dreamer pinned to the wall of my room. I felt it was a remarkably poetic statement, and so true to my own life, and it summed up much of my own philosophy on human existence:

It doesn't interest me what you do for a living.
I want to know what you ache for,
And if you dare to dream of meeting your heart's longing.
It doesn't interest me how old you are.

I want to know if you will risk looking like a fool
For love
For your dreams
For the adventure of being alive.

It doesn't interest me what planets are squaring your moon.
I want to know if you have touched the centre of your own
    sorrow,
If you have been opened by life's betrayals,
Or become shrivelled and closed
From fear of further pain.

And so it goes on. There are thirteen verses in all, and one speaks of being 'faithless, and therefore trustworthy'. To me the meaning here was all about love. It was about not clinging to rigid dogmas or beliefs to the exclusion or derogation of all others, about being non-judgemental. And the last verse really, really touched me.

I want to know if you can be alone
With yourself
And if you truly like the company you keep
In the empty moments.

After the first sixteen years of my dark and abusive life I reckoned I was just starting to reach the stage where I could be alone with myself and like who I was 'in the empty moments'. I hoped Tom did too.

One day I found Tom reading 'The Invitation' intently. Once he was done he turned to me and said, 'Wow! You're deep!'

I looked at him. 'I hope so. I've lived too much to be shallow.'

It wasn't long after that that I started to tell Tom some of what had happened to me as a child. I feared doing so, for I feared that Tom might run. But if I didn't tell him, and if I didn't reveal all, then I felt our relationship would be based upon a lie. And if it was, when he told me he loved me it wouldn't be the real me that Tom was loving.

So Tom had to know. Like Samantha, if Tom was my true soul mate he wouldn't turn away from me and leave. He would accept me, damaged and bruised and full of life's betrayals as I was. If after hearing it all, Tom would still 'risk looking like a fool for love', then he was the one for me.

Telling Tom everything was difficult, but it was also cathartic and truly liberating. Tom is a gentle, caring soul, with untold hidden strengths and a huge heart. Exactly one year after we met, Tom proposed to me. It was Christmas Eve, 2007, and we were at midnight mass at St Bride's Church once again. He asked me if I would marry him.

I barely hesitated before saying: 'Yes! I will!'

The vicar announced the happy news of our engagement there and then, and there was a spontaneous round of applause, and cheering. I smiled inside myself. I had finally said yes to 'Oddball Tom'. Tom finds it funny that that's how I used to think of him. He tells a very different story of our getting together. The way he tells it, he's more like the knight in shining armour!

Maybe it's possible for a person to be both. I think it is. I think he's my knight in shining armour too.

Chapter Twenty-seven

Lavender Dreams

Perhaps because of finding Tom, and finding love, I felt strong enough within myself to try to make contact with my family again. They had never once apologised for what they had done to me. They had simply issued accusations about what I had done to them: dishonouring my father, and besmirching the family name. Even so, I still wanted to know them, if I possibly could. They were my family, and I would never get another one.

But it wasn't to be. I did manage to make contact with my youngest sister, Aliya. She and I had always got on well, and she'd never been such the goody-goody, perfect Muslim daughter that Sabina, the older of my two younger sisters, had been. I hoped I might find some common ground with her. We made a little stilted small talk before I got down to saying what I wanted to say.

'I could come to visit you,' I suggested. 'I could bring my flatmate, Samantha. She's really nice. You'd like her.'

Aliya sounded horrified. 'How could you do that to Mum and Dad? After all that you've done, you're trying to bring a dirty gori infidel into this house!'

'I'm also a "dirty infidel",' I countered. 'So where does that leave us?'

'Yes, I suppose you are . . . You're unclean, like the rest of them. In fact, I doubt if I'd even want to be in the same room as you.'

The conversation didn't last a lot longer than that. I was shocked and appalled. My little sister had always been so much more the mellow one of my siblings. But in the time that I had been away the blind prejudice and hatred of my father had seeped into her veins. How could it have happened? It was all so messed-up and so sad.

To make matters worse, I received a text message shortly after that, from Raz.

Get this: you'd better come back to Islam. Come back to Islam right now. Unless you do, you are apostate: I will not be responsible for my actions.

I could hardly believe that I had received such a message from my gentle brother Raz – he who had escorted me to school to receive my English prize, all those years ago. I knew the experience in the Pakistani madrassa had scarred him deeply, but this was a new and frightening side of Raz's character.

None of my brothers had been in that knife-wielding mob that my father had raised to kill the 'traitor' – me. I had never expected any of them to take up the campaign of hatred that Dad had started and make it their own. But now it seemed that Raz was on the path towards doing so. Poor Raz. Dad really had succeeded in damaging him.

For now at least it was clear that there was no way back to my family. I was grief-stricken by their response. It was like losing them all over again. Was I surprised that they were still so entrenched in their ways? Not really. But if I'm honest with myself I had always nurtured a flame of hope that we might be reconciled. Now that flame had been extinguished.

The principal act that had made me so abhorrent to my family was my leaving Islam – my apostasy. I had had the temerity to believe that I had the right to choose my own faith, to follow my own belief system, to listen to my own heart.

All the reasons they had for turning against me were so wrong. They believed I had been wrong to flee my family; in fact, I had every right to do so. They believed I had been wrong to defy my father's will: I had every right to do so. They believed I had been wrong to avoid a forced marriage: again, I had every right. They believed I was wrong for choosing my own belief system; yet I had the right. *I had the right.*

That last, to me, seemed the least of my 'sins'. But to my family and my community, it was the ultimate betrayal.

As for me, I felt they were rejecting the very person I had become. For the first time in my life I thought that I was a good person to know. I had started to believe in myself. I had so much to offer other people: my friends, my work colleagues, and now my fiancé. Yet my family were still trying to reject and deny all of that – to bury me in that dark place where they had imprisoned me for so long.

I felt that I had much to offer to people that I didn't know – through my work, speaking at communities, youth groups, charities, and the workshops. In that context, my life was a bridge between two worlds, two belief systems and two cultures that were increasingly finding themselves at war with each other. There was so much conflict, distrust and misunderstanding, but I knew and understood both sides. I had experienced both sides and *lived* them.

I understood what was needed to help bring both sides closer together, and to break down the barriers of distrust and enmity. It was never going to be easy: the fear, prejudice and ignorance ran deep. But it was work – a mission – that I truly believed in. And it was a message that I dearly wanted my family to hear. But it seemed that they were absolutely, resolutely closed to my every single word.

I did go to the police to report Raz's threats. And they did take it seriously. Certain measures were put in place to protect me. The saddest thing was that I had to move out of the house that I shared with Samantha. I couldn't countenance putting her in danger.

When I was nineteen years old I had bashed out a few small fragments of my life story on a battered little typewriter. It was interspersed with several awkward poems in which I tried to express my hurt, my betrayal and pain. I wasn't in any sense writing my life story. I was just trying to help myself understand what had happened to me by putting it down on paper.

As a child I had written diaries and little stories. As a nineteen-year-old I hoped writing might help me to understand and better deal with how I was feeling. I thought that my poems were embarrassing and rubbish. But however badly worded and clumsily rhymed they were, they did express how I was feeling at the time, and they helped me come to terms with my dark past.

There was one that I entitled 'Inside My Mind'. I was twenty-one years old when I wrote it. I read it now, and it's not so bad:

Inside My Mind

Inside my mind there lives,
Dreams of lives I could have lived,
With You inside of me
Holding me, beside me.
But first I have to let
You catch my thoughts in your net.
To take away my dirt,
My pain, my hurt.
Then I hope I can forgive,
And live and love and give.
Help me, Oh Lord, to be
The Father's child you see in me.
I need You to heal me, let
You catch my thoughts in your net.
To take away my dirt,
My pain, my hurt.
I wish, I wish I could
Be the Father's child You would,
If he'd not stolen all my love,
Filled me with lies and mud.
He took my caring heart,

My love, my childish part,
My innocence, my golden mind,
And filled it with all the filth he could find.

There are a series of recurring themes in these poems – confusion and betrayal over past darkness, and the quest to be free. Here's one that I entitled, simply, 'Free'. It's not exactly very good, but does communicate how I was feeling at the time:

Free

I've got to be free again.
Free to fly into the sky,
Like a bird flying,
I've got to be free.
I've got to be free again.
Free to say what I want,
Free to be what I want,
I've got to be free.
I've got to be free again.
Free to love and trust,
Free to be and trust,
I've got to be free.
I've got to be free again.
Free from a world of fear and pain,
Free like the wind,
I've got to be free.
I've got to be free again.
Free to be whoever I want to be,
Free to discover the real me,
I've got to be free.

After a while I stopped the writing. I had realised that I had a habit of getting too into it, and becoming a recluse. I would get lost in the story, not speaking to people for days on end. This was similar to what I had done as an abused child, when I had constructed my make-believe world of the Loneliness Birds and the Lavender Fields. I had retreated to that world whenever my physical presence had been beaten and abused, in the dark cellar.

I stopped the writing and began instead speaking at schools and churches about my life, trying to communicate a lesson to others. I remember a little school kid once asked me: 'Why are you brown? Did God make you brown?'

It was a good question. Why was I brown? I didn't feel very 'brown' at the time, or rather I didn't feel very happy within my skin – for me it signified all the troubles from which I had fled. In fact, back then I wished I'd been born into a white English family. If I had been, the first sixteen years of my life might not have been so horrible, and full of darkness and betrayal. At least, that's what I told myself back then.

These days, I'm very happy with my colour. I wouldn't wish it any other way. Tom and I got married in the spring of 2008, and we will, I hope, go on to have cappuccino-coloured kids. I just know they're going to be beautiful.

The wedding itself was a dream-like affair. We were wed at St Bride's Church, and all my friends and surrogate families were there. Rachel and Samantha were my bridesmaids. Felicity and James travelled down from Bermford, to help give me away. Tom, his best man and the ushers wore matching top hats and tails, with a single white rose in their buttonhole. Tom looked gorgeous in his black jacket and charcoal grey trousers, his crisp white shirt and lavender cravat. For once I realised what a seriously handsome man I had netted in Tom!

Lavender was the theme colour for the wedding. The church, the invitations, the flowers and even the napkins and tablecloths at the reception were decorated with lavender butterflies. Down the central aisle of the light and airy church were tethered lavender-coloured balloons, each decorated with butterflies, plus our names – Hannah & Tom. My own dress was a classic white strapless number, and I wore a single diamond nose stud, plus a tiara in my hair.

As for my bridesmaids, they each wore a dress the same

gorgeous hue of lavender. I have rescued lavender from the fields of my dreams as an abused child, and made it my colour. For me it now signifies love, life and hope. And for me the butterfly has become a metaphor for my transformation – out of darkness into the light.

The church was packed with friends and relatives. They'd volunteered to decorate the church, cook the food, take the photos and video, and do just about anything else they could think of to keep the costs down. Samantha's father led me down the aisle, as Tom waited for me at the altar to say 'I do'. I was late, of course, and Tom was a bag of nerves by the time I got there. His best man had been teasing him remorselessly that I'd had a last-minute change of heart!

I hadn't changed my mind. There were no last thoughts. I gazed happily into Tom's eyes and I did say, 'I do'. And then Tom was allowed to kiss the bride. A huge cheer went up from the hall as Tom trapped me in an enthusiastic embrace, and a kiss that just seemed to go on and on and on. Tom always does seem to have his own special way of doing things.

After we had tied the knot, there was a reception in the church hall upstairs. Jenny – the one person most responsible for getting Tom and me together – had offered to provide the music. She sings with a husky, slinky, chocolate-spiced voice that sends shivers up my spine every time I hear it. She sang 'Summertime' for us, whilst we stood at the top of the stairs and welcomed all our friends and relatives and thanked them for being there for us on our special day.

> *Summertime . . .*
> *And the livin' is easy.*
> *Fish are jumpin'*
> *And the cotton is high.*
> *Oh your daddy's rich*
> *Your ma is good lookin',*
> *So hush, little baby*
> *Don't you cry.*

One of these mornings
You're gonna rise up singin',
Then you'll spread your wings
And you'll take to the sky.
But till that mornin'
There's a nothing can harm you
With daddy and mammy standin' by.

Meeting and now marrying Tom was the summertime of my life. I had found my way to the sunshine and the light. And with Felicity and James being there at my wedding, I had my other mum and dad with me – those who had rescued me and first taken me out of the darkness. And in Samantha and her parents I had my second surrogate family, those who had welcomed me to a place where I could finally lay to rest the threat of vengeance from my family. I owed them all so much. I owed them my life and my happiness.

After the wedding reception, I was whisked away by Tom on a surprise honeymoon. It was the loveliest of surprises for me when, after a long flight, we touched down on sun-washed, glistening white tropical sands in a place close to paradise.

Tom is a tender and gentle soul, and I've been blessed in finding him. As Felicity had promised me when I was sixteen and had just run away, I had finally met the man of my dreams and fallen in love. And being physically intimate with Tom didn't unsettle me at all.

I am happy with my religion and my identity now. But for every girl born a British Muslim who, like me, manages to escape, there are many more that do not. Many remain trapped in *forced* marriages – as opposed to arranged marriages – and abusive relationships, living a life little better than slavery.

Of course, there are lots of Muslim women in Britain who live full and liberated lives. But I know personally of too many who are imprisoned in marriages to men brought over from rural

Pakistan who drink, and beat and rape them. Their husbands believe that the Quran justifies all of this abuse. They believe that their wives are their property, to be used as they see fit. Of course, there are many Muslim marriages that are good ones. I use the phrase 'forced' marriage, as opposed to arranged marriage, to denote a girl married by force and against her will.

I meet such women via the charities I work with. Very little seems to have changed since I was in that situation. In some cases it actually seems to be getting worse. However, some local authorities have set up advice centres solely for women. There are places where Muslim women can find people to talk to. They have a chance to find out what their rights are, and to discover that what is being done to them is wholly wrong, and illegal under British law. There are some refuges for women, but many, many more are needed.

I met one Bangladeshi family through my work with Crossways. The entire family had converted from Islam to Christianity: the mum, the dad, four girls and one ten-year-old boy. The community had put huge pressure on them to return to Islam. Eventually, they couldn't hold out any longer, and half the family converted back again. The little boy and the youngest daughter stayed with the parents. But the oldest three girls – twenty-one, eighteen and sixteen years old – were determined to carry on being Christians.

These three girls knew they were in grave danger. They decided they needed to get away from their community, and they rang me. I phoned around some refuges, but none seemed willing to take them because they hadn't actually been physically attacked. I was appalled. What was the point of waiting until the damage had been done before offering help? If those girls had been attacked by a forty-strong mob, as I so nearly was, what was the chance that they would be as lucky as me, and escape? By then the injuries, *or the killing*, would have been done – and they would need a hospital or a morgue, not a refuge.

Fortunately, I was able to locate a family in another town who were willing to look after the three Bangladeshi sisters for a few days. We would have to see where they might go from there. But there is a crying need for shelters where people in such situations can find refuge, and escape the kind of life-and-death situations that had faced me in my teens, and now faced those three sisters, and others like them.

At that time there had been a lot of coverage in the newspapers about apostasy, especially the dangers faced by women who leave Islam. I read those articles and wonder whether those women ever got any help. And then there are the girls fleeing from forced marriages; the women who commit suicide to escape their husbands; the parents who kill their own daughters, because they have somehow 'dishonoured' them.

One case in particular stuck in my mind. A teenage Muslim girl was forced to drink bleach by her uncle and brother, before being stabbed to death by them. Her crime? Refusing an arranged marriage. Her mother was present when she was murdered, and seemingly did nothing to stop it. It was so horrific, I could barely read that story without feeling physically sick. A dark chill went through me. I knew that it was a case of – *there but for the grace of God went I.*

In London there is a sizeable Moroccan Muslim community. A number of the women had secretly converted to Christianity, but in public they remained Muslims. Otherwise, their husbands and family would threaten to take their children away, and worse. They were forced to lead a double life, behaving as good Muslims in public, and sneaking into churches whenever they could. And this in a country that supposedly guarantees people the right to pursue their beliefs – or lack of them – freely, as they desire.

I have worked with organisations that deal with the Moroccan community, teaching women English and helping them to better establish their lives. I've spoken with women forced to lead this double life; Islamic in name, but sneaking into churches when they can. Some just give up their right to pursue their beliefs freely as they so desire – for the dangers and risks associated with the double life are extreme.

But where is the freedom of worship in all of this? The United Kingdom is one country that espouses religious freedom, and freedom of belief is supposed to be a fundamental human right. But where is it in practice, especially amongst the British Muslim community?

And this is not only about choosing one faith or another: it is equally unacceptable to many Muslims to leave Islam *and choose no faith at all.* Leaving Islam to become an atheist is just as abhorrent, if not more so, and attracts the same censure and danger. There isn't even the freedom *to choose not to believe.*

What struck me so strongly was that no one ever seemed willing to talk about this, or go public on it. It is rarely in the press, because the media doesn't have access to such stories. There is little or no debate at the political level. Most organisations working in this field stay silent. Their priority is to retain access to these women in very difficult and challenging circumstances. Speaking out won't help them do so, and they know it. Silence is the only practical option.

But if that conspiracy of silence continues unchallenged, nothing will ever change. Where is the outcry? Where are the defenders of human rights, women's rights and religious rights, crying out for justice? Instead, I hear regularly of 'honour killings' taking place in the UK, and what a lie that phrase is! Time after time I hear of girls suffering the same fate as almost befell me. I hear of girls taking their own lives, rather than submitting to the cruel indignities that their parents, and their culture, thrust upon them.

And these are only the tip of the iceberg. For all the cases that make it into the courts, or the press, how many more are covered up and silenced? Imagine how easy it would have been for my father to ship me off to Pakistan and get me married off. Imagine how simple it would have been to have me dealt with – by murder if necessary – had I resisted. Imagine how the community would have closed ranks and protected him, throwing a blanket of silence over the disappearance of his daughter.

I escaped from an Asian Muslim ghetto, but only by the skin

of my teeth. Far from everything is bad about the culture, the belief system, and the community that I left. There is much of great value there: community cohesion and spirit; respect for elders; a strong sense of identity; a sense of values informing modesty and good behaviour. In fact, there are aspects of the community and family I left behind me that I still miss. But there is also much that needs breaking down, building up again, and mending.

It is for those reasons that I decided to speak out. That is why I decided to take the risk and break the silence.

Chapter Twenty-eight

Silence Broken

One day I had a phone call from one of the charities that I worked with. They explained that there was a TV documentary being made about arranged marriages, by Channel 4, one of Britain's foremost broadcasters. Would I be willing to be interviewed?

At first, I was hesitant. I had no idea what it might entail. But I agreed to see the producer for a chat. We met in a café, in Paddington Station. She was a young white woman, and she seemed to know exactly what she was doing. The feeling I got from her was that she would do everything in her power to protect me, if I agreed to participate in the film.

She made it clear that I could pull out at any moment if I didn't feel safe and secure. She had drawn up a contract guaranteeing to protect my identity, and agreeing not to show my face on screen, or anything else that might identify me. She won my confidence, and eventually I agreed to be interviewed for the film.

It took a whole day to shoot the interview. It was done in London, and lots of scenes were filmed with me walking down the street and around the local park. I was only shown from behind, the camera concentrating on my feet or my hands – parts of me that revealed nothing of my identity.

I spoke in my real voice, and that wasn't going to be disguised. I reckoned that I had been away from the north of England for long enough for me to have soaked up a southern accent. My voice had changed so much that I figured no one would recognise it, not even my close family.

The interviewer was a different woman from the producer that I had met. She asked me about my life story and why I ran away from home. I spoke about fleeing a forced marriage, about converting out of Islam and the 'crime' of apostasy. I spoke about going on the run and being forced into hiding. I talked about the mob and the death threats. But I told them nothing about the deeper issues that lay behind my escape.

'Are there other girls in this situation?' the interviewer asked.

'Yes, obviously,' I replied. 'A lot of young Muslim women are suffering as I did.'

'What can be done to help them?'

'There's a real need to understand the challenges posed by Islamic culture,' I said. 'We need to provide escape routes for girls like me, because they are horribly trapped where they are right now. And we need to start talking about it. We need to open a debate. We need to get it into the open. Silence doesn't help. It makes it worse, in fact.'

It was a bit odd being under those harsh TV lights. But I enjoyed the filming and meeting the production team. They seemed to be a lovely, caring bunch, and entirely professional. What was more, I thought it was very important work that they were doing. I felt it was crucial for people to hear what I, and other victims and survivors, had to say. We could speak for so many other women entombed within a dark, unbreakable silence.

I left the interview feeling as if I had done the right thing. I asked if they could show me a rough edit of what they were going to put in the programme, before it was broadcast. They invited me up to London again, and the producer lady gave me a DVD to watch on my computer. What I saw reassured me that my identity was protected. It was that more than anything that I wanted to reassure myself about.

The programme broadcast a few weeks after the filming. I was really happy to have been part of it. I watched it at home with Samantha and Chris. Both of them were pleased for me, and proud that I had had the guts to speak out.

After that broadcast, more requests started coming in for interviews, usually via the same charity. I agreed to do an interview over the phone for a Sunday morning show on BBC radio. Then there was a call from a journalist with a flagship current affairs TV programme. They were making a film about converts from Islam and the issue of apostasy, and how such converts were treated in this country.

I talked to the film's producer. He told me it was all but impossible to find people who were willing to speak, even anonymously, about apostasy. One Pakistani Muslim family had agreed to do so. They hailed from my own home town. After their conversion they had been attacked on the streets, and their church had been besieged by a violent mob. The film makers had got hold of CCTV footage of much of this actually happening. I agreed to do an interview, but only if my identity was disguised.

Then, in the autumn of 2007, I met Josephine, a British religious freedom campaigner. We happened to be at a networking meeting in London, together with charities that work within the Muslim community. Josephine was there to advise on how to get such stories out into the media, without compromising the brave men and women who were willing to speak out.

I gave a brief presentation regarding my own experiences. I explained what I was doing with my own charitable work, especially the workshops I was holding for young Muslim women. Afterwards, Josephine came up and introduced herself. We met up later for a coffee and a chat and we soon struck up a friendship. Over time, I told Josephine some of my story.

Josephine was about to launch a new religious freedom charity, based in London. She asked me if I would attend the launch at the Frontline Club, a private members' club in West London set up for and by war reporters. It was invitation-only, so I felt fairly safe attending. But I was concerned as to what it would be like, for I had never been to such an event before.

I arrived at the Club early, at Josephine's request. She had asked if I might speak privately with one or two journalists who would be there. In no time several of them were trying to talk to me all at once. Finally, Josephine interrupted in her very schoolmarmy way.

'No, no, no!' she smiled, but with a steely look in her eye. 'Poor Hannah. All of you at once! We can't have this. You'll have to take it in turns.'

I breathed a sigh of relief. That made a lot more sense. First I spoke to a journalist from *The Times*. Josephine told the next reporter he had to buy me lunch, because I hadn't eaten yet. So his interview took place in a curry house across the road from the Club. After that I was too tired to do any more, but I did agree to do the remainder of the interviews by phone.

I told the journalists my story of fleeing a forced marriage, my conversion out of Islam, and being hunted by my family for so many years. I mentioned nothing of the darker pain and betrayal and abuse. I spoke about the concept of apostasy and what it means. It all seemed an absolute eye-opener for them. They were visibly shocked. How, they asked me, could such things be happening on the streets of Britain in the twenty-first century?

How indeed.

After that, Josephine received a flood of requests for media interviews. I agreed to a few of them. But eventually, I had to call a halt. It was taking over my life, and I still had my work to do.

But I did agree to one more, with one of the BBC's major radio programmes. Josephine said it was important, because the show was listened to by so many people. She took me to the BBC studio to do the interview. The interview was perfectly fine, but towards the end the reporter chose a form of words that seemed – rightly or wrongly – to question my motives for being there.

'So what do you hope to achieve by speaking out?' she asked. 'Surely, you'll just cause more trouble?'

What a stupid question. Was she trying to suggest that I should keep quiet so as not to cause any 'trouble'? And if so, how was that supposed to help the young girls and women trapped in situations like the one from which I had escaped? Was silence going to help them? Wasn't causing some 'trouble' exactly what was needed? How much good had the years of silence done all the young women facing violence, forced marriage and worse? What had silence and submission ever achieved for them?

I was angered by the thrust of her question. It seemed to me to be informed by misguided political correctness, mixed with a good dose of ignorance. I had recently read a book by Arthur Koestler, the author and sometime philosopher. One phrase from it stuck in my mind: 'The predicament of Western civilization is that it has ceased to be aware of the values which it is in peril of losing.' It was written at the time in reference to communism, but remains as relevant today regarding the rise of a particular kind of prejudiced, uninformed Islam – the sort of Islam as espoused by my father.

To me, that journalist's question was part of a larger mis-apprehension that plagues Western civilisation – that if we simply ignore it and don't cause any 'trouble' it might all just go away. The sort of problems that darkened the first sixteen years of my life will *never* simply go away. Now more than ever we need to stand up for the values and freedoms that we in Britain, and the rest of the free, democratic world, cherish: freedom of expression, freedom of political choice, and freedom of belief.

The remarks of that journalist were like a red rag to a bull. Rather than keeping quiet so as not to cause any trouble, *trouble I was going to cause*. I was going to keep speaking and speaking and speaking out.

It was then that I decided that this book had to be written. I dug out the yellowed, typewritten pages that I had composed when I was nineteen years old. As I read them over, fragments of a past life, and of the dark horrors and the escape, came rushing back to me. Memories piled upon memories. Now, where was I to start?

I don't remember much from when I was little. The images are sketchy, dull smudges amongst the shades of grey. But I do remember my street. My street was good fun. It was great on my street.

Epilogue

This is my story and I have told it as accurately as my memory allows. Sometimes, the way we remember events is different from the way others do, and I apologise if I have made any significant errors in my story's telling. In my eyes my life is not about misery: it is about love. The philosopher Sophocles once said; 'One word frees us of all the weight and pain of life: that word is *love*.' That is what I believe.

I was a caged butterfly, but I have flown free from what some would call the ghettoised Muslim community, but what I would call the trap of uninformed Islam. I seized hold of my freedom: freedom to choose what I believe; freedom to speak out about my beliefs; freedom to live a life as I see fit, even when others don't agree. I am a free woman in a world where there are many women encaged.

I am not the only woman who has thus grasped my freedom. There are others who have chosen to leave Islam, and therefore have become *murtadd* – apostates. This is a story dedicated to them, too. Jesus Christ once said: 'I have told you these things, so that in me you may have peace. In this world you will have trouble. But take heart! I have overcome the world' (John 16:33). I took heart. I seized the moment, and I seized my right to be free. Others can too. You only have to take the first, and the most difficult, step.

In much of my life I felt fear that held me back from living, but I believe we, all of us, can live a life without fear and at peace with ourselves, and others. As I look at this world, again and again I see fear: the politically correct fear of offending Muslims; the fear of Islamist terrorism; the fear Muslims have that they will all be branded as 'terrorists'. We need to overcome this corrosive, vicious cycle of fear that breeds on fear. And the starting point of doing so is breaking the silence.

As Ayaan Hirsi Ali says, in her book, *Infidel*: 'People ask me if I have some kind of death wish, to keep saying the things I do. The answer is no: I would like to keep living. However, some things must be said, and there are times when silence becomes an accomplice to injustice.' I am inspired by such people to speak out about what I believe to be true. Dr Martin Luther King once said; 'Our lives begin to end the day we become silent about things that matter.' I believe absolutely that I must speak out, and I believe absolutely that we can find ways to live together with those who are different from ourselves, without fear.

I cannot be silent about what happened to me, and what is still happening to countless other young girls and women today. Of course, my own experiences were made worse by the fact that my father was a particularly abusive man. In that respect, his religion was irrelevant. But it is also true that some of the abuse I suffered was made all the more damaging because it was tolerated silently by my family and my community, in as much as they knew about it. This was very much a result of my culture and echoes the experience of other Muslim women I have met and read about.

This leads me to be concerned for the future of the Muslim community in this democratic country, and democratic countries around the world. I am worried for Muslim women who, like me, want to choose to live a free life in Britain, across Europe, in the USA and elsewhere, but cannot because of the straightjacket of 'honour' and 'shame' that controls many of them, and the entrenched attitudes of some of the communities that they inhabit.

Belief is a uniquely personal thing. Freedom to believe as the individual sees fit – or not to believe for that matter – is a defining feature of civilisation. If we no longer have the willingness or strength to defend people's freedom of choice in religion, then we have lost the very foundations of our civilisation. And that way, intolerance and totalitarianism lies.

Since writing this book I have spoken out widely about my story and the wider issues it raises. In the UK, the USA and elsewhere I have talked to gatherings of 5,000-plus people at a time. It was at first a daunting prospect, but I do this because I cannot be silent about injustice. And I shall keep doing so because I love life, and I love my fellow humans who inhabit this world.

> I leave you peace, my peace I give you . . .
> so don't let your hearts be troubled or afraid.
> John 14:27

Appendix

All direct Quranic quotations and commentary in this book are taken from *Interpretations of the Meanings of the Noble Quran, with Commentary*, translated by Dr Mohammad Taqi-ud-Din Al-Hilali and Dr Muhammad Muhsin Khan.

The Quranic quotes used in this book are:

Page 9: 'Do not with your own hands cast yourselves into destruction,' Surah 2:195

Page 9: 'Do not kill yourselves,' Surah 4.29

Page 30: 'O you who believe! Do not take the Jews and Christians for friends; they are friends for each other; and whoever amongst you takes them for a friend, then surely he is one of them.' Surah 5:51; also, in other places, it includes altogether more positive comments about them. Surah 5-82.

Page 91: the Quran says quite clearly that menstruation is an 'indisposition', and that menstruating women are 'unclean'. Surah 2:222

Page 213 and 226: anyone who converts away from Islam and refuses to return should be killed. Surah 4:89

Page 225: there was a chapter entitled 'Women', about how Muslim women should be treated. Surah 4.

Page 225: husbands were allowed to 'beat' their wives for 'ill-conduct'. Surah 4:34.

Page 225: a wife was 'tilth' for her husband. Surah 2:223.

Page 226: Jesus – a healer. Surah 3:49.

Page 226: in the Old Testament it said that Abraham was asked to offer up his son, Isaac, for sacrifice. In the Quran, he is asked to offer up Ishmael. Surah 37:102–109.

Page 229: the Quran upholds modest dress. Surah 24:31.

Page 230: the very word Islam means 'submission'. Surah 2:45.

Page 230: the Quran does speak of being a 'slave of Allah'. Surah 9:93.

The Hadith source (referred to on Page 213) is taken from www.usc.edu/dept/MSA/fundamentals/hadithsunnah/bukhari and is translated by Sahih Bukhari, *Volume 9, Book 84, Number 57*:

Narrated 'Ikrima:

Some Zanadiqa (atheists) were brought to 'Ali and he burnt them. The news of this event, reached Ibn 'Abbas who said, 'If I had been in his place, I would not have burnt them, as Allah's Apostle forbade it, saying, "Do not punish anybody with Allah's punishment (fire)." I would have killed them according to the statement of Allah's Apostle, "Whoever changed his Islamic religion, then kill him." '